Understanding Lung Cancer

A Guide for Patients

Dr. Mrityunjay Sharma
Dr. Deepanjali Sharma

Dedication

To our parents, for your unwavering love, support, and wisdom. This book is a testament to your enduring legacy. With deepest gratitude and love.

Contents

Chapter 1: The Human Respiratory System 1

Anatomy of the Respiratory System 1

Physiology of the Respiratory System 4

Other Functions of the Respiratory System...................... 7

Impact of Lung Cancer on the Respiratory System......... 10

Chapter 2: Cancer and Its Types................................ 12

Cell Growth and Division:.................................... 12

What Goes Wrong in Cancer? 14

Tumour Development and Spread........................ 16

Types of Cancer 17

Chapter 3: Classification of Lung Cancer...................... 23

Non-Small Cell Lung Cancer (NSCLC) 23

Small Cell Lung Cancer (SCLC)............................. 25

Other Types of Lung Cancer 26

Rationale for Classification................................ 26

Benefits of Classification................................ 27

Primary and Secondary Lung Cancers..................... 29

Chapter 4: Causes and Risk Factors 31

Smoking and Secondhand Smoke 31

Environmental Factors................................. 32

Workplace exposure................................. 33

Outdoor air pollution 34

Genetic factors 34

Previous Lung Disease 35

Infections................................. 35

Chapter 5: Clinical features of Lung Cancer 37

Signs and Symptoms 37

Paraneoplastic Syndromes 40

Chapter 6: Diagnosis 42

Medical History 42

Physical Examination 44

Role of Imaging in Lung Cancer Diagnosis 46

Advanced interventions 49

Role of Biopsy in Diagnosing Lung Cancer 52

Non-Invasive Diagnostic Tool 55

Histopathological and Molecular Analysis 55

Chapter 7: Lung Cancer Staging 59

TNM Classification System 59

Staging of Small Cell Lung Cancer (SCLC) 62

Chapter 8: Screening for Lung Cancer 64

Chapter 9: Treatment Lung Cancer 67

Treatment Overview 67

Surgery 69

Types of Resection Techniques 70

Radiation Therapy 73

Types of Radiation Therapy 73

Chemotherapy 76

Types of Chemotherapy 76

Side Effects of Chemotherapy 83

Targeted Therapy 87

Types of Targeted Therapy 89

Immunotherapy 91

Types of Immunotherapies 91

Chapter 10: Palliative Care in Lung Cancer 95

Strategies for Effective Palliative Care Implementation
.... 97

Chapter 11: Prehabilitation and Rehabilitation for Lung
Cancer 100

Chapter 12: Living with Lung Cancer 105

Lifestyle adjustments 105

Financial and Legal planning 108

Chapter 13: Prevention of Lung Cancer 110

Chapter 14: The Future of Lung Cancer Research and
Treatment 116

Advances in Early Detection and Screening 116

Emerging Therapies 118

Preface

Lung cancer is one of the most challenging diseases, affecting millions of people worldwide. This disease has become the most common cause of cancer-related deaths globally. Typically, the late presentation of this disease makes its management more difficult. The journey through lung cancer diagnosis, treatment, and recovery is often fraught with uncertainty, fear, and many questions. Being doctors, we have had the privilege of working closely with such patients. We have witnessed that the unawareness and lack of knowledge about the disease's development and its causes have led to more suffering and poorer outcomes. However, we have also witnessed the incredible resilience of people. This book is born out of those experiences and our desires to provide a comprehensive resource for everyone, including patients, their families, and caregivers.

The primary goal of this book is to empower you with knowledge. Knowledge about what lung cancer is, what the causes are, how it is diagnosed, screening for early identification, and the various treatment options available. Understanding these aspects can help you remove the causative factors from your life and prevent the disease as much as possible. Additionally, understanding different aspects of the disease will help you make informed decisions and feel more in control during a challenging time. We have also discussed the latest advancements in lung cancer research and treatment to offer hope and insight into what the future may hold.

While no book can cover every aspect of lung cancer, we have endeavored to include the most relevant and up-to-date information. This includes sections on prevention strategies, early detection, personalized treatments, and supportive care. This guide also extends to the emotional and psychological challenges that come up with the lung cancer diagnosis, providing strategies for coping and maintaining a positive outlook.

This book is intended for anyone affected by lung cancer—patients, loved ones, caregivers, and even those seeking to understand the disease better. We will start with an introduction to the respiratory system, its anatomy & physiology, and then followed by detailed chapters on causes, risk factors, signs & symptoms, prevention, early detection, and various treatment modalities. Special sections are dedicated to the future of lung cancer research and living with lung cancer, offering a holistic view of managing the disease.

Our hope is that this book will serve as a valuable companion, offering both information and encouragement. Remember, you are not alone on this journey. With the right knowledge, support, and care, it is possible to prevent, as well as navigate lung cancer with hope and determination.

Thank you for choosing this guide. We wish you a happy and healthy life ahead.

Dr. Mrityunjay Sharma

Dr. Deepanjali Sharma

Disclaimer!

The information provided in this book is for educational and informational purposes only. It is not intended as a substitute for professional medical advice, diagnosis, or treatment. Always seek the advice of your physician or other qualified healthcare providers with any questions you may have regarding a medical condition.

Do not disregard professional medical advice or delay seeking it because of something you have read in this book. The authors, publishers, and contributors of this book are not responsible for any adverse effects or consequences resulting from the use of any suggestions, preparations, or procedures discussed in this book.

Lung cancer is a serious and complex disease that requires individualized medical treatment and care. This book is not intended to be used for self-diagnosis or self-treatment of lung cancer or any other health condition. If you suspect you have lung cancer or have been diagnosed with it, you must seek care from qualified healthcare professionals.

Medical knowledge and practices are constantly evolving, and new information may emerge that could change the recommendations or information presented here. Therefore, readers are encouraged to consult with their healthcare providers to obtain the most up-to-date information and guidance.

Chapter 1: The Human Respiratory System

The respiratory system is one of the most vital organ systems in the human body and is responsible for carrying out the process of respiration (breathing). The process of respiration has two phases: inspiration (inhalation) and expiration (exhalation). During the inspiratory phase, air goes into the lungs, where a gaseous exchange between the lungs and blood takes place, and consequently, oxygen is delivered to the bloodstream. In the expiratory phase, air comes out of the lungs along with the waste product of metabolism, carbon dioxide. In order to keep this whole process of respiration smooth and continuous, all the components of the respiratory system, whether structural or functional, work in great synchrony. So, before we begin to learn about lung cancer, how it develops, how it affects breathing, and overall health, understanding the basic structure (anatomy) and function (physiology) of the respiratory system is crucial.

Anatomy of the Respiratory System

The respiratory system can be divided into the upper and lower respiratory tracts. The upper respiratory tract starts from the nose and continues up to the voice box, which is also known as the larynx. The anatomical structures or parts the upper respiratory tract includes are the external orifices of the nose, the cavity behind them (the nasal cavity), the throat (also known as the pharynx, which is the common area behind where the nasal cavity and the oral cavity meet with each other), and the voice box (also known as the larynx, responsible for sound production). The lower respiratory tract begins just after the larynx and extends up to the alveoli. Structures included in the lower respiratory tract are the windpipe (also known as the Trachea, which is the largest airway), the medium and small airways (also known as the Bronchi and the Bronchioles, respectively), and the alveoli (sac-like microscopic structures responsible for gas exchange). (Fig. 1.1 and 1.2)

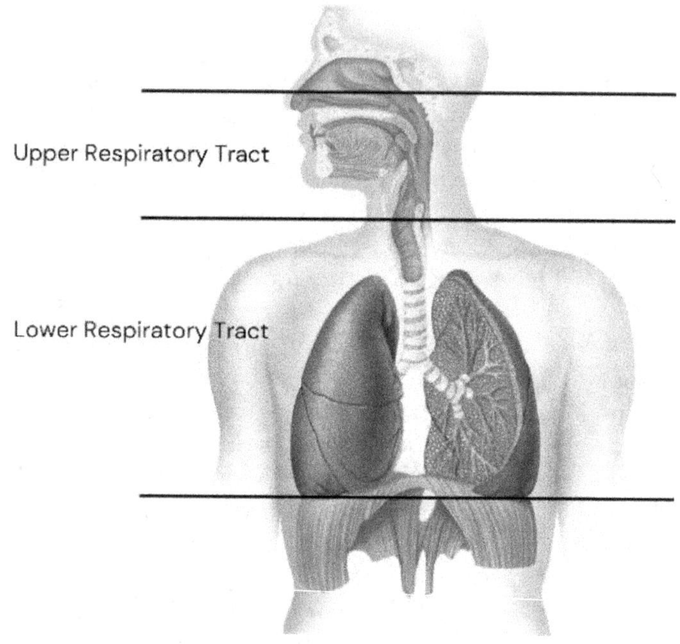

(Fig. 1.1: Upper and lower divisions of the respiratory tract)

Upper Respiratory Tract:

- **Nose and Nasal Cavity:** The primary entrance for outside air. The nasal cavity has a zigzag bony structure covered with mucosa within it, which warms, filters, and humidifies the air coming in through the external nasal openings, also known as external nares.

- **Pharynx (Throat):** This is comparatively a larger space behind the nasal cavity that serves as a pathway for air moving from the nasal cavity towards the larynx. The pharynx also serves as the pathway for food coming from the oral cavity towards the esophagous, which is the food pipe situated behind the windpipe (trachea).

- **Larynx (Voice Box):** Located below the pharynx, the larynx contains the vocal cords for sound production and acts as a narrow passageway for air between the pharynx and trachea.

Lower Respiratory Tract:

- **Trachea (Windpipe):** This is a 12 cm long hollow tube-like structure for the passage of air. The trachea consists of C-shaped cartilaginous rings that keep it open and prevent its collapse during expiration or more severe actions like coughing (Fig. 1.2).

- **Bronchi and Bronchioles:** The lower part of the trachea divides into two branches known as primary bronchi (one bronchus for each lung). The bronchi are relatively smaller in size and width than the trachea. The bronchus of each lung further subdivides into smaller branches known as bronchioles. These bronchioles extend into the lobes of the lungs and create a branching network within the lungs (Fig. 1.2).

- **Alveoli:** The bronchioles, after reaching the lobes of the lungs, keep on dividing into smaller branches, and after numerous divisions, they reach the deepest part of the lungs to open into the small sac-like structures known as alveoli. These alveoli are microscopic structures and are surrounded by a network of very small and thin-walled blood vessels, known as capillaries, for the gaseous exchange between the alveoli and the blood circulated within the capillaries (Fig. 1.3 and 1.4).

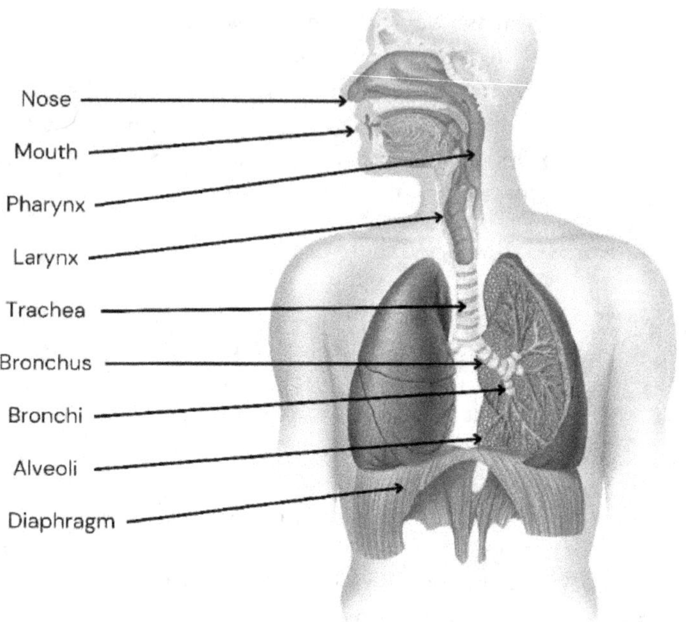

(Fig. 1.2: Anatomical Structures of the Respiratory System)

Physiology of the Respiratory System

Role of the Lungs in Gas Exchange

The primary responsibility of the respiratory system is to supply oxygen (O_2) and remove carbon dioxide (CO_2) from the blood stream through the process of gas exchange. This exchange takes place between the alveoli and the blood in the capillaries across the alveolar-capillary membrane. There are millions of alveoli present in human lungs, and together they form a vast surface area for efficient gaseous exchange across their thin walls. (Fig. 1.3). During inhalation, oxygen reaches the alveoli, which results in a high partial pressure of oxygen within them. The capillaries surrounding the alveoli have blood, which has been coming after circulation in the whole body. During circulation, the oxygen from the blood is utilized by the cells of the body. This consumption of oxygen leads to a low partial pressure of oxygen in the blood, also known as deoxygenated blood. Since the capillaries surrounding the alveoli have this deoxygenated blood and have a low partial pressure of oxygen, a pressure difference is built between the alveoli and the capillaries surrounding them. This pressure difference results in the diffusion of oxygen from high pressure (within alveoli) to low pressure (within capillaries). After diffusion into the blood, oxygen binds with hemoglobin in red blood cells (forming oxyhemoglobin) and then circulates in the whole body through the blood stream.

Simultaneously, the exact opposite happens with carbon dioxide. During circulation, carbon dioxide, which is the byproduct of metabolism, gets released into the blood from cells. The increased amount of carbon dioxide leads to a high partial pressure of carbon dioxide in the blood. Since the capillaries surrounding the alveoli have this deoxygenated blood with high partial pressure of carbon dioxide, diffusion of carbon dioxide from high pressure (within capillaries) to low pressure (within alveoli) takes place. After diffusion into the alveoli, carbon dioxide is expelled from the body through exhalation (Fig. 1.4).

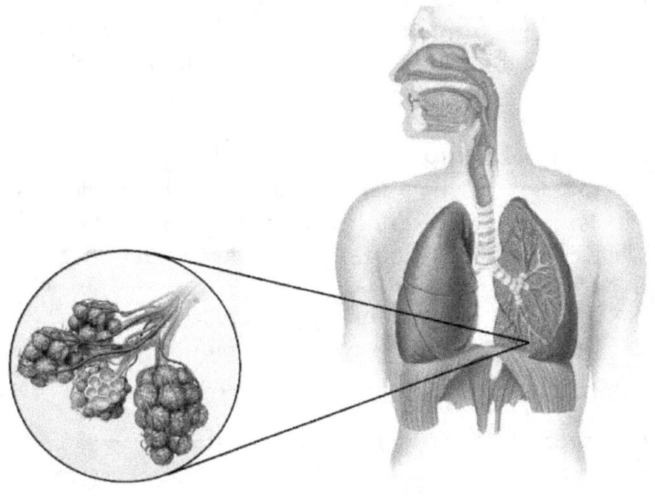

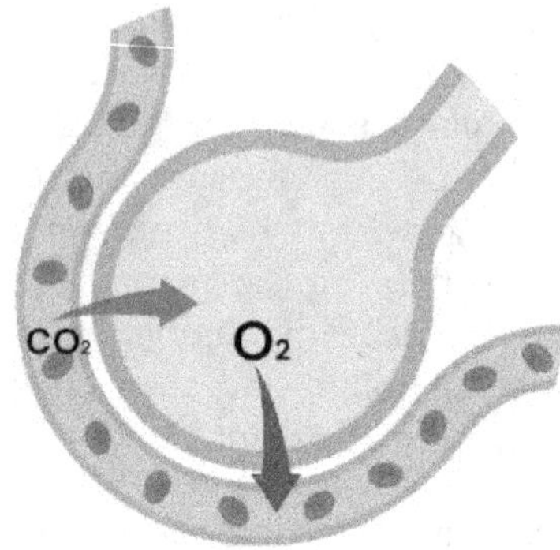

(Figs. 1.3 and 1.4 show an expanded view of alveoli surrounded by capillaries and a simplified version of the same to illustrate the exchange of O2 and CO2 between alveoli and blood capillaries, respectively.)

Phases of Respiration

1. Pulmonary Ventilation (Breathing): The movement of air into and out of the lungs is known as pulmonary ventilation. It involves two phases: inhalation (inspiration) and exhalation (expiration). The diaphragm and the muscles of the thorax, for example, intercostal muscles and pectoralis major muscles help in expanding and contracting the thoracic cavity during the inspiration and the expiration, respectively.

2. External Respiration: The exchange of oxygen and carbon dioxides between the alveoli and the blood in the capillaries. Oxygen diffuses from the alveoli into the blood, while carbon dioxide diffuses from the blood into the alveoli.

3. Transport of Respiratory Gases: Oxygen binds with hemoglobin and the oxygenated blood circulated in the whole body within the circulatory system.

4. Internal Respiration: When the oxygenated blood reaches the tissues of the body, an exchange of gases takes place between the blood and the body's tissues. Oxygen diffuses from the blood into the cells, and carbon dioxide diffuses from the cells into the blood.

Other Functions of the Respiratory System

In addition to its primary role in gas exchange, the respiratory system performs many other wide range functions, which are essential and vital for overall health and the maintenance of homeostasis. These functions include:

1. Regulation of Blood pH

The pH is a unit, which is essentially used to measure the acidity or the alkalinity of something. The pH of the human body ranges from 7.35 to 7.45. Maintenance of this range of pH is paramount for all the enzymes in the body to work properly. A derangement in the pH, either low or high, is very dangerous for life. The levels of pH are maintained by the levels of CO_2 and bicarbonate (HCO_3) in the blood. So, as you know by now, the respiratory system's primary function, to help exchange gases, also regulates the levels of carbon dioxide (CO_2) in the blood, which eventually balances the pH in the blood. If the pH of the body increases or decreases, the respiratory system changes its pace and depth of respiration to accumulate or remove more CO_2 from the blood in order to decrease or increase the pH, respectively. This adjustment brings the pH level back to normal and within range. Thus, the respiratory system also plays a crucial role in regulating the body's acid-base balance.

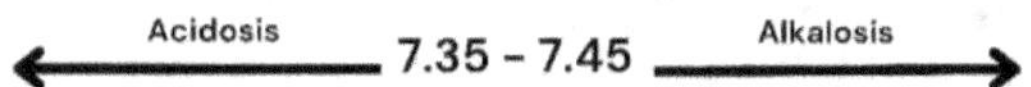

A decrease in blood CO_2 levels is the consequence of hyperventilation, which is defined as fast and deep breathing, which causes an excess exhalation of CO_2. Reducing carbon dioxide levels leads to a change towards alkalosis, particularly respiratory alkalosis, because carbonic acid and bicarbonate form a buffer system in the blood. On the other hand, carbon dioxide retention leads to elevated blood levels in hypoventilation, which is marked by shallow and slow breathing. When carbon dioxide levels are high, the concentration of carbonic acid rises, causing a drop in blood pH and respiratory acidosis. In both cases, the changes in CO2 levels and, by extension, blood pH, show how breathing patterns affect acid-base homeostasis.

2. Vocalization

When it comes to producing voice and speaking, the respiratory system is absolutely essential. Vocal cords are housed in the larynx, also known as the voice box. During exhalation, the vocal cords vibrate due to the air passing through the larynx, which in turn produces sound. Changing the amount of airflow by increasing or decreasing the flow of air by the lungs and the tension in the vocal cords allow one to alter the pitch of the sound pitch and its volume.

3. Olfaction (Sense of Smell)

Chemicals in the air can be detected by olfactory receptors located in the nasal cavity. The epithelium (a thin layer of tissue that covers organs, glands, and other structures) that covers the nasal cavity is known as the olfactory epithelium. This olfactory epithelium contains receptors for olfaction. During the process of inhalation or exhalation, when air crosses the olfactory epithelium, odorant molecules get attached to the olfactory receptors, and in turn, the receptors send signals to our brain to sense and interpret the smell.

4. Protection and Filtration

The respiratory system protects us from harmful particles, for example, dust or pathogens. There are several mechanisms for this purpose:

- Mucociliary clearance: The lining of the respiratory tract is covered with mucus and fine, hairlike structures known as cilia. When harmful particles come into the airway with air, they get trapped in the mucus. The cilia of the respiratory epithelium move in a synchronized fashion to move the mucus upwards and towards the throat. Once the mucus reaches the throat, it is either spitted out or swallowed.

- Cough Reflex: This is another highly protective reflex that clears the airways of irritants or any foreign particle by forceful expulsion.

- Nasal Hairs: The nasal cavity contains small, fine hair that acts as a filter to entrap unwanted particles from the inhaled air.

5. Thermoregulation

The respiratory system helps regulate body temperature by conditioning the air that is inhaled. The rich blood supply in the nasal cavity warms the air before it reaches the lungs.

6. Metabolic Functions

The lungs are also involved in some of the enzymatic processes vital for life beyond gas exchange. These processes include the synthesis, activation, and inactivation of certain enzymes.

- **Conversion of Angiotensin I to Angiotensin II**: The enzyme angiotensin-converting enzyme (ACE), located in the pulmonary endothelium, converts angiotensin I to angiotensin II, a potent vasoconstrictor involved in blood pressure regulation

7. Blood Reservoir

This pulmonary circulation serves as a reservoir for blood. At a time, approximately 10% (500 ml) of the body's total blood volume remains in pulmonary circulation. This 500 ml of blood acts as a reservoir and helps maintain adequate cardiac output and systemic blood pressure.

Impact of Lung Cancer on the Respiratory System

The impact of lung cancer on the system is significant. It disrupts the functioning of the lungs, affecting parts such as the bronchi, bronchioles, and alveoli.

1. Airways Blockage: Tumours may grow in the bronchi or bronchioles leading to complete blockage. This can cause breathing difficulties, wheezing and a persistent cough.

2. Lung Tissue Damage: Cancer cells can invade lung tissue reducing its ability to efficiently exchange gases. This could result in lower oxygen levels in the blood.

3. Pleural Effusion: Lung cancer might lead to fluid accumulation in the pleural space. Lungs are covered by a membrane called the pleura. There are two layers of pleura: the inner one is called the visceral pleura, and the outer one is called the parietal pleura. Pleural space is the space between these two layers of pleura. When fluid gets accumulated in this space, it compresses the lungs, causing chest pain and breathing problems.

4. Metastasis: Cancer has the property to spread (metastasize) to other parts of the body. Due to this property, lung cancer in one lung can spread to any part of the respiratory system, for example, the other half of the lung, nearby lymph nodes, etc. This can further spread to other organ systems as well, for example, organs and blood vessels situated in the mediastinum, the diaphragm, the chest wall, the liver, brain, bones, etc. Due to this metastasis, lung cancer

not only affects the primary site but also affects the overall respiratory function and general health.

5. Secondary Infections: Blocked airways due to tumour compromise ventilation and the ability of the lung to clear secretion. These complications compromise lung function as well as predispose the respiratory system to harbour secondary bacterial infections.

Chapter 2: Cancer and Its Types

Cancer is an intricate and diverse illness that can impact any region of the body, causing disturbances in regular bodily processes and presenting substantial health challenges.

Definition of Cancer

Cancer is defined as a group of diseases characterized by the uncontrolled division and spread of abnormal cells. The cancerous cells have a property to spread to other places and form tumours there as well. These cells invade nearby tissues or spread to other parts of the body through the blood and lymphatic systems. This complete process of spread is called metastasis.

Cell Growth and Division:

- **Cell Cycle:** The cell cycle is a continuous ongoing process in the human body by which cells undergo continuous growth and division. The cells cycle also replace the old or damaged cells. The cell cycle comprises distinct stages, namely growth, DNA synthesis, preparation for division, and cell division. Cell cycle is a very complex process, and there are uncountable components of it that help to run the cycle smoothly. For example, there are some DNA-protein structures located at the end of our chromosomes, which are responsible for protecting the chromosome's integrity throughout the cell cycle.

- **Cell cycle checkpoints:** The cell cycle is closely controlled by checkpoints that ensure cells undergo division only when they are in a healthy state and under appropriate conditions. Checkpoints function as monitoring systems, temporarily halting the process to mend DNA damage or verify the exact replication of all cellular components prior to cell division. In the context of cancer, these regulatory mechanisms are frequently evaded or compromised, resulting in unrestricted cellular growth.

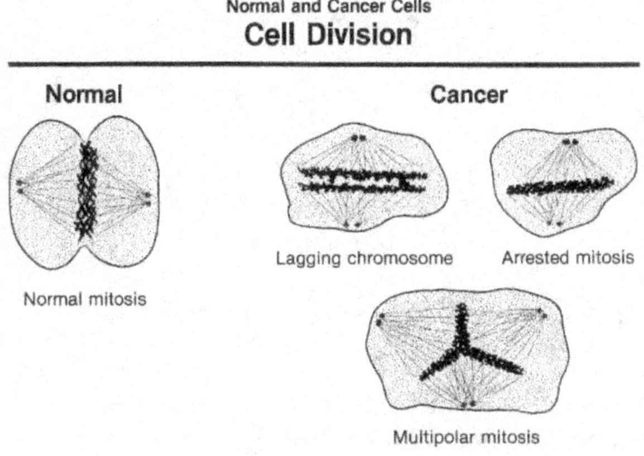

Fig. 2.1: This image compares normal cell division to abnormal division in cancer cells. In normal cell division (normal mitosis), chromosomes align correctly and are evenly distributed into two new cells. However, in cancer cells, division often goes wrong. There can be lagging chromosomes that don't separate properly, arrested mitosis where the division process stops incorrectly, or multipolar mitosis where more than two spindle poles form, leading to an uneven distribution of chromosomes. These errors result in genetic instability, which contributes to the uncontrolled growth characteristic of cancer. (Source: National Cancer Institute; Creator: Pat Kenny)

DNA and Genes:

- **DNA:** DNA, the genetic material, contains the instructions for all biological processes and is organized into genes. DNA is a helical molecule consisting of nucleotides, and it contains the necessary instructions for the growth, operation, and reproduction of all living species.

- **Genes**: Genes are precise DNA sequences that encode proteins, which are the primary molecules responsible for carrying out various biological activities. Genes govern the production of proteins that regulate the cell cycle, repair defective DNA, and manage cell death (apoptosis). Genetic mutations in these specific genes can result in the development of cancer either by triggering the synthesis of atypical proteins or by inhibiting genes that suppress tumour growth.

What Goes Wrong in Cancer?

Cancer occurs when this normal regulation breaks down, leading to uncontrolled cell growth. Here are the key concepts in cancer biology simplified:

1. **Mutations**: Changes or errors in the DNA.

    - **Causes**: Mutations can be caused by various factors, including:

        - **Environmental Exposures**: Such as tobacco smoke, UV radiation, and certain chemicals.

        - **Inherited Mutations**: Passed down from parents.

        - **Random Errors**: Occurring during cell division.

2. **Oncogenes, Tumour Suppressor Genes, and DNA Repair Genes**:

    - **Oncogenes**: Normal genes that, when mutated, become permanently activated and promote excessive cell growth.

- **Tumour Suppressor Genes**: Genes that normally slow down cell division or cause cells to die at the right time. To simplify this concept, imagine oncogenes as a gas pedal and tumour suppressor genes as the brakes on a car. In a cancer cell, the gas pedal is stuck down (mutated oncogenes), and the brakes have failed (mutated tumour suppressor genes). The car speeds out of control, ignoring all signals to stop.

- **DNA Repair Genes:** Genes responsible for repairing DNA damage. When these genes are mutated, cells accumulate genetic damage more quickly, which can lead to cancer.

3. **Hallmarks of Cancer**: Key characteristics that differentiate cancer cells from normal cells:

   - **Sustaining Proliferative Signaling**: Cancer cells keep signaling themselves to grow and divide, even when they shouldn't.

   - **Evading Growth Suppressors**: They ignore signals that would normally stop their growth.

   - **Resisting Cell Death**: Cancer cells avoid the usual process of programmed cell death (apoptosis), which removes damaged or unnecessary cells.

   - **Enabling Replicative Immortality**: Normal cells can only divide a limited number of times, but cancer cells can keep dividing indefinitely.

- **Inducing Angiogenesis**: They stimulate the formation of new blood vessels to supply the growing tumour with nutrients and oxygen.

- **Activating Invasion and Metastasis**: Cancer cells can break away from their original site and spread to other parts of the body.

Tumour Development and Spread

1. Tumour Formation: A tumour is the result of an uncontrolled cell division that begins with a single mutated cell. This process initiates when the regulatory mechanisms that typically regulate cell growth and division malfunction, frequently as a result of genetic mutations.

- **Benign Tumours:** Benign tumours are non-cancerous growths that do not disseminate to other regions of the body. They are typically encapsulated, which means they are confined within a well-defined boundary, and they tend to develop slowly.

- **Malignant tumours:** These cancerous growths have the potential to invade adjacent tissues and disseminate to remote regions of the body. They are not encapsulated, which enables them to infiltrate surrounding tissues, and they tend to proliferate more rapidly.

2. Metastasis: The process by which cancer cells disseminate from the primary site to generate new tumours (secondary tumours) in other regions of the body.

- **Invasion**: Cancer cells invade nearby tissues.

- **Intravasation**: Cancer cells enter blood vessels or lymphatic vessels.

- **Circulation**: Cancer cells travel through the bloodstream or lymphatic system.

- **Extravasation**: Cancer cells exit blood vessels to invade new tissues.

- **Colonization**: Cancer cells establish new tumours in distant organs.

Cancer is a result of changes in the DNA that disrupt the normal regulation of cell growth and division. These changes allow cells to grow uncontrollably, evade death, and spread to other parts of the body.

Types of Cancer

Cancer can arise from nearly any cell or organ system within the body. The categorization, or nomenclature, of the cancer type is typically determined by the specific cellular or tissue origin. It is crucial to identify and comprehend various types of cancers in order to effectively treat them, as each cancer type possesses distinct characteristics.

1. Carcinomas

Carcinomas are the most common type of cancer. They originate in the cells of epithelium, which line the surfaces of organs of the body. They are classified on the basis of histology (the study of the microscopic structure of tissues).

- **Adenocarcinoma**: Forms in mucus-secreting glands and is common in cancers of the breast, colon, and prostate.

- **Squamous Cell Carcinoma**: Arises in the squamous epithelium, often found in the skin, lungs, and esophagus.

- **Basal Cell Carcinoma**: A type of skin cancer that originates in the basal cells of the epidermis.

- **Transitional Cell Carcinoma**: Develops in the urinary system, including the bladder, ureters, and renal pelvis.

2. Sarcomas

Sarcomas arise from connective and supportive tissues of the body. Connective tissue is defined by tissue that connects, protects, supports, and gives structure to other organs system in the body. Examples of connective tissue are bone, cartilage, fat (adipose), muscle, and blood. Sarcomas can be classified into the following categories.

- **Osteosarcoma**: The most common type of bone cancer, typically occurring in the long bones of the arms and legs.

- **Chondrosarcoma**: Cancer of the cartilage.

- **Liposarcoma**: Cancer that begins in fat cells.

- **Leiomyosarcoma**: Cancer of smooth muscle tissue, often found in the uterus, gastrointestinal tract, or blood vessels.

- **Rhabdomyosarcoma**: Cancer of skeletal muscle tissue, more common in children.

3. Leukemias

Cancer can develop in the blood and the bone marrow (soft tissue withing bones that produces blood). Leukemias are cancers characterized by the uncontrolled production of abnormal white blood cells in the blood and bone marrow.

- **Acute Lymphoblastic Leukemia (ALL)**: Rapidly progressing leukemia that affects immature lymphoid cells.

- **Acute Myeloid Leukemia (AML)**: Rapidly progressing leukemia affecting myeloid cells.

- **Chronic Lymphocytic Leukemia (CLL)**: Slowly progressing leukemia affecting lymphoid cells.

- **Chronic Myeloid Leukemia (CML)**: Slowly progressing leukemia affecting myeloid cells.

4. Lymphomas

Lymphomas are cancers that originate in the lymphatic system, which is part of the immune system. The lymphatic system is an intricate network of thin vessels. These vessels extend throughout the body. The system of lymphatics facilitates the removal of fluid, known as lymph, from the tissues and returns it to the bloodstream. Lymph nodes Lymph nodes are the bean shaped structures present in the body. They serve as filters for lymph transported by lymphatic system. Lymph nodes house lymphocytes (a type of white blood cell) that aid in the body's defence against infection and disease.

- **Hodgkin Lymphoma**: Hodgkin lymphoma is a cancer of the lymphatic system. It is characterized by the presence of Reed-Sternberg cells. It typically begins in the lymph nodes and can spread to other organs as well.

- **Non-Hodgkin Lymphoma**: A diverse group of cancers that include any kind of lymphoma except Hodgkin's lymphomas. In Non-Hodgkin lymphoma malignant cells are formed in the lymph system. They originate in lymphocytes and can be further classified into B-cell or T-cell lymphomas.

5. Myeloma

Myeloma is a cancer that originates in the plasma cells of the bone marrow. Plasma cells are a specific type of leukocyte (white blood cell) produced in bone marrow. They originate from B lymphocytes (B cells). When plasma cells encounter bacteria and viruses, they produce antibodies in order to combat them and prevent disease.

- **Multiple Myeloma**: The most common type of myeloma, characterized by the accumulation of abnormal plasma cells in the bone marrow, leading to bone damage and affecting blood cell production.

6. Central Nervous System Cancers

The central nervous system includes the brain and spinal cord.

- **Gliomas**: There are a variety of cells in the brain. A group of tumours that start in glial cells are called Gliomas. There can be more types, for example, astrocytomas, oligodendrogliomas, and ependymomas.

- **Meningiomas**: Tumours that form in the meninges, the protective membranes covering the brain and spinal cord.

- **Medulloblastomas**: Commonly occurring in children, these tumours start in the cerebellum, which controls balance and coordination.

7. Germ Cell Tumours

Germ cell tumours originate from the cells that give rise to sperm or eggs. These tumours usually occur in the ovaries or testes, but they can also develop in other parts of the body.

- **Testicular Cancer**: Most testicular cancers are germ cell tumours.

- **Ovarian Germ Cell Tumours**: They develop in the ovaries and are typically found in younger women.

8. Neuroendocrine Tumours

These tumours originate from neuroendocrine cells, which have traits of both nerve cells and hormone-producing cells.

- **Carcinoid Tumours**: These are slow-growing tumours and are usually found in the gastrointestinal system or lungs.

- **Pancreatic Neuroendocrine Tumours**: These are the tumours that arise from the hormone-producing cells of the pancreas.

9. Melanoma

Melanoma is a type of skin cancer that originates in melanocytes. Melanocytes are the cells which are responsible for producing melanin. Melanin is the pigment that gives skin its color.

- **Cutaneous Melanoma**: The most common type, occurring on the skin.

- **Ocular Melanoma**: Melanoma that develops in the eye.

- **Mucosal Melanoma**: Melanoma occurring in the mucous membranes of the body, such as the nasal passages, throat, and vagina.

Cancer is a diverse group of diseases with various types classified based on their origin in different cell types and tissues. Each type of cancer has unique characteristics, treatment approaches, and implications for patient health.

Understanding these distinctions is crucial for effective diagnosis, treatment, and management of cancer.

Chapter 3: Classification of Lung Cancer

Lung cancer encompasses a range of diseases originating from epithelial cells. Proper classification of lung cancer plays a role, in diagnosing, treating, predicting outcomes and advancing research. This section will explore the categorization and various forms of lung cancer the criteria for classification and the advantages it offers. Broadly speaking lung cancer can be categorized into two types: Non-Small Cell Lung Cancer (NSCLC) and Small Cell Lung Cancer (SCLC). This initial classification is determined by the appearance of tumour cells. It is essential for guiding subsequent treatment plans and predicting prognosis.

(Note: Histological appearance is the representation of the microscopic structure and organisation of cells and tissues as they are observed through a microscope. This appearance is a consequence of the complex arrangement of cells, extracellular matrix, and other components that constitute the tissue. The comprehensive insights into the cellular morphology and tissue architecture that histological appearance provides are essential for the identification and diagnosis of a variety of diseases, including cancers.

Non-Small Cell Lung Cancer (NSCLC)

The majority of lung cancer cases, around 85%, are classified as non-small cell lung cancer (NSCLC). This type is divided into three categories: adenocarcinoma, squamous cell carcinoma and large cell carcinoma. Recognizing these subtypes is essential for the diagnosis, treatment and management of lung cancer.

Adenocarcinoma

Adenocarcinoma is the form of lung cancer particularly among individuals who do not smoke. It originates from the glandular cells in the lining of the lungs and typically develops in the outer regions of the lungs.

Key features

- Histology: Examination under a microscope shows glandular patterns and mucin production. The cells may create structures resembling glands and produce mucus.
- Epidemiology: Adenocarcinoma is more frequently detected in women and younger patients.
- Etiology: Non-smoker risk factors may include mutations, exposure to radon gas, asbestos and air pollution.

Squamous Cell Carcinoma

Squamous cell carcinoma originates from the cells that line the airways and is commonly located in the regions of the lungs, near the main bronchus.

Key features

- Histology: The histological traits of this cancer type include the formation of keratin (a protein found in skin and hair). These cells resemble the squamous cells found in the skin and mucous membranes.
- Epidemiology: This particular lung cancer is more prevalent among men and older individuals.
- Etiology: There is a strong association of squamous cell carcinoma with smoking. The harmful substances in tobacco smoke directly harm the cells lining the airways and cause this cancer.

Large Cell Carcinoma

Large-cell carcinoma is a less common yet more aggressive form of non small cell lung cancer (NSCLC). It lacks the characteristic features of large and squamous cells, as are seen in adenocarcinoma and squamous cell carcinoma.

Key features

- Histology: Large cell carcinoma showcases large, undifferentiated cells that lack specific structural differentiation.

- Epidemiology: Both smokers and non-smokers can be affected by this type though its exact prevalence patterns are not well known.

- Etiology: Although smoking is a known risk factor, the specific causes of cell carcinoma are not as clearly defined as for other NSCLC subtypes.

Small Cell Lung Cancer (SCLC)

Small cell lung cancer (SCLC) accounts for about 15% of all lung cancer cases. It is distinguished by its rapid growth and early metastasis. It often spreads to distant body sites before even symptoms appear. This type is almost exclusively associated with smoking. Due to its rapid progression and metastasis, SCLC is considered as an aggressive cancer that requires prompt and intensive treatment.

Key Features

- Histology: SCLC is characterized by small, round, and densely packed cells. These cells have scant cytoplasm, finely granular chromatin, and absent or inconspicuous nucleoli. The tumours often exhibit a high mitotic rate (high-rate cell division) and areas of necrosis (death of tissue due to absent blood supply).

- Epidemiology: SCLC is strongly linked to people who smoke heavily. It is rare among non-smokers and more common in men.

- Etiology: The primary risk factor for SCLC is smoking. The carcinogens in tobacco smoke cause genetic mutations that lead to uncontrolled cell division and development of SCLC. Other potential contributing factors besides smoking include exposure to secondhand smoke, radon gas, asbestos, and other environmental toxins.

Other Types of Lung Cancer

Besides the major types of NSCLC and SCLC, there are several other less common forms of lung cancer. Each of them has their unique characteristics and implications for treatment.

Adenosquamous carcinoma contains the features of both the adenocarcinoma and the squamous cell carcinoma. The dual nature of these types makes it challenging to diagnose and treat.

Sarcomatoid carcinoma is a rare and aggressive subtype of lung cancer that includes both epithelial and sarcomatous elements.

Carcinoid tumours are a type of neuroendocrine tumour that arises from the hormone-producing cells of the lung. These cancers are generally less aggressive than small cell lung cancers. Carcinoid tumours are classified into typical and atypical carcinoids.

Mesothelioma is a rare and aggressive cancer that primarily affects the lining of the lungs (pleura) and is almost exclusively linked to asbestos exposure.

Rationale for Classification

The classification of lung cancer into NSCLC and SCLC, and further subtypes, is not arbitrary. It is based on several important factors:

Histopathological Differences

Histological examination of tumour tissues reveals distinct cellular patterns and features, which are used to categorize lung cancer. This microscopic evaluation helps in identifying the origin and differentiation of the cancer cells.

Molecular and Genetic Profiles

Recent advances in molecular biology have shown that different types of lung cancer have unique genetic mutations and molecular signatures. For example:

- EGFR mutations are commonly seen in adenocarcinomas.

- KRAS mutations are also frequent in adenocarcinomas but rare in squamous cell carcinoma.

- ALK rearrangements are another hallmark of certain adenocarcinomas.

Clinical Presentation and Behavior

Different types of lung cancer present differently in terms of symptoms, growth rates, and patterns of metastasis. For instance:

- SCLC is known for its rapid growth and early metastasis.

- Adenocarcinomas often metastasize to distant organs like the brain and bones.

Therapeutic Implications

Treatment strategies vary significantly between different types of lung cancer. For example:

- SCLC is typically treated with chemotherapy and radiotherapy due to its aggressive nature.

- NSCLC may be treated with surgery, targeted therapy, immunotherapy, or a combination, depending on the stage and molecular characteristics.

Benefits of Classification

Classifying lung cancer into specific types has numerous benefits for patients, clinicians, and researchers.

Improved Diagnosis and Staging

Accurate classification allows for precise diagnosis and staging, which are crucial for determining the appropriate treatment plan. It also helps in identifying the prognosis and potential outcomes for the patient.

Personalized Treatment Plans

With the advent of precision medicine, treatments can be tailored based on the specific type and genetic profile of lung cancer. For example:

- Targeted therapies such as EGFR inhibitors or ALK inhibitors are used for adenocarcinomas with specific mutations.

- Immunotherapy has shown promise in treating various forms of NSCLC with high PD-L1 expression.

Enhanced Prognostic Accuracy

Different types of lung cancer have different prognoses. For instance:

- SCLC generally has a poorer prognosis due to its aggressive nature.

- Adenocarcinoma patients with early-stage disease and specific mutations may have a better prognosis with targeted therapies.

Facilitation of Research

Classifying lung cancer helps in the design of clinical trials and research studies. Researchers can focus on specific subtypes to develop and test new treatments, improving the overall understanding of the disease.

Better Patient Management

Clear classification aids in patient management, including monitoring for recurrence, managing side effects, and providing supportive care. It ensures that patients receive the most appropriate and effective care based on their specific type of lung cancer.

Primary and Secondary Lung Cancers

There are two categories of lung cancer: primary and secondary. It's important to distinguish between these types for a diagnosis and tailored treatment plan.

Primary lung cancer originates in the lungs itself. The two primary types are Non Small Cell Lung Cancer (NSCLC) and Small Cell Lung Cancer (SCLC). NSCLC, being more common accounts for around 85% of cases. It includes subtypes like adenocarcinoma, squamous cell carcinoma and large cell carcinoma. In contrast SCLC is less common but more aggressive. Treatment for lung cancers depends on their characteristics and often involves a mix of surgery, chemotherapy, radiation therapy as well as advanced treatments, like targeted therapy and immunotherapy.

On the hand, secondary lung cancer does not originate in the lungs but spreads there from another part of the body. These cancers maintain the characteristics of the tissues they originated from.

Cancer that spreads to the lungs, from parts of the body like breast, colorectal, prostate, kidney or melanoma can lead to lung cancer. Treating lung cancer involves dealing with the cancer and controlling its spread. This usually involves treating the cancer and using treatments, like chemotherapy, targeted therapy or immunotherapy.

Lung cancer can be classified into two broad categories: primary and secondary lung cancers. Understanding the difference between these types is crucial for accurate diagnosis and appropriate treatment.

Key Differences Between Primary and Secondary Lung Cancers

Aspect	Primary Lung Cancer	Secondary Lung Cancer
Origin	Begins in the lung tissue itself	Spreads to the lungs from another primary site in the body
Diagnosis	Diagnosed through imaging, biopsies, and identifying lung cancer type	Involves identifying the primary cancer site through imaging and biopsies
Treatment	Focuses on the lung cancer itself, using surgery, chemotherapy, radiation, targeted therapy, and immunotherapy	Directed at the primary cancer and its metastases, often involving systemic treatments like chemotherapy, targeted therapy, or immunotherapy
Prognosis	Varies based on type and stage; generally, better for NSCLC than SCLC	Dependent on the primary cancer type and extent of metastasis
Common Types	NSCLC (adenocarcinoma, squamous cell carcinoma, large cell carcinoma), SCLC	Breast cancer, colorectal cancer, prostate cancer, kidney cancer, melanoma

By understanding these distinctions, patients and healthcare providers can better navigate the complexities of lung cancer diagnosis and treatment. While primary lung cancer is focused on the lungs themselves, secondary lung cancer requires a broader approach, addressing both the original and metastatic sites to effectively manage the disease.

Chapter 4: Causes and Risk Factors

There are several causes and risk factors that can cause lung cancer. An understanding of these causes and risk factors can help prevent lung cancer or detect it early. This chapter will discuss the causes and risk factors of lung cancer to reveal how genetics, lifestyle choices, and environmental factors can cause it.

Smoking and Secondhand Smoke

Smoking is the leading cause of lung cancer, accounting for about 85% of all cases. The chances of developing lung cancer increase sharply with an increase in the number of cigarettes smoked. Cigarettes contain agents that can cause cancer, called carcinogens. When burned, cigarettes create more than 7,000 chemicals. At least 70 of these chemicals are known to cause cancer.

Secondhand smoke, also known as passive smoke or environmental tobacco smoke, is the smoke from a burning tobacco product or the smoke exhaled by a smoker. Nonsmokers breathe many of the same carcinogens as smokers do. Living with a smoker increases a nonsmoker's risk of developing lung cancer by 20-30%. Secondhand smoke exposure occurs in the home, in cars, and at work, when tobacco products are consumed. It is especially more hazardous for children, pregnant women, and persons with preexisting health concerns. Passive smoking increases the risk of heart disease, stroke, lung cancer, and respiratory infections.

Pack years:

The term "pack-years" is used in medical communities to measure the period a person has been exposed to tobacco. In this way, it provides a standardized perspective on the hazards associated with smoking diseases such as lung cancer, chronic obstructive pulmonary disease (COPD), and heart attack.

The calculation of pack-years is simple:

Formula:

Pack-years=(Number of packs of cigarettes smoked per day) × (Number of years smoked)

Example:

If a person has smoked 1 pack of cigarettes per day for 20 years, the calculation would be:

Pack-years = 1 pack/day × 20 years=20 pack-years

The number of packs of cigarettes smoked per day is calculated using a common unit of measurement i.e. one pack equals twenty cigarettes. So, if a person smokes 20 cigarettes every day, it equals one pack per day. When someone smokes ten cigarettes a day, it is referred to as 0.5 packs per day. The number of years smoked is the total number of years for which a person has smoked. It is critical to include smoking exposure duration, regardless of whether there were any breaks or variations in how strongly and frequently the person smoked. The pack-years calculation is useful not only for determining the level of tobacco smoke exposure, but it also has practical applications in both clinical and research settings. The number of pack years provides an idea of the amount of exposure and the risk of developing smoking-related diseases, for example, chronic obstructive pulmonary disease (COPD), lung cancer, etc. Based on a high number of pack years, physicians may categorize the person into high-risk groups for screening.

Environmental Factors

Radon is a radioactive gas produced by the natural decay of uranium in rocks and soils, and it may additionally be detected in water. It is not possible to sense the presence of this gas in our surroundings with our natural senses since it is an odourless, colourless, and tasteless gas. Usually, Radon seeps from the ground and decays into radioactive particles, which can be inhaled and cause DNA damage, which can potentially lead to lung cancer. In outdoor areas where proper ventilation is present, the levels of radon are usually low. However, indoors, especially in poorly ventilated areas like mines and caves, levels can be much higher. The level of radon is measured in Bq/m^3. The high level of radon poses a significant risk to the people who are exposed to it. As per the data from different sources, radon has been identified as the second most common cause of lung cancer after smoking, responsible for around 3% to 14% of total lung cancer cases. Radon enters buildings through various openings and is usually higher in basements. Since the levels of radon may fluctuate within buildings depending upon the area they are situated in and ventilation, a regular measurement of the radon level is advisable. Effective methods to reduce radon include improved ventilation, radon sump systems, sealing floors and walls, and using radon ventilation fans. In drinking water, radon is more prevalent in groundwater sources. Inhalation of this gas poses a greater risk than ingestion. There are a few techniques, like aeration and granular activated carbon filters, that can reduce the levels of radon in water supplies.

Workplace exposure

Workplace exposure to the following carcinogens increases the risk of lung cancer significantly: Asbestos and other cancer-causing substances such as respirable crystalline silica, nickel, chromium (VI), and polycyclic aromatic hydrocarbons (PAHs) are some of the most common carcinogens at the workplace. Mining and the use of asbestos in industries such as construction, shipyards, and manufacturing pose significant risks. Exposure to arsenic in wood preservatives, pesticides, and electronics, as well as exposure to beryllium in nuclear and aerospace technologies, increases lung cancer risk. Workers in the nickel and chromium industries get exposed to carcinogenic agents during metal processing. Similarly, silica dust, especially in mining and construction, and polycyclic aromatic hydrocarbons in aluminum and rubber manufacturing are significant contributors to lung cancer risk.

Outdoor air pollution

Outdoor air pollution is a combination of small dust-like particles and several other elements that might influence health. Burning coal or wood and smoke from factories and vehicles are the main sources of outdoor air pollution. Though smoking still greatly increases the risk factor, research indicates that outdoor air pollution is responsible for approximately 1 in 10 cases of lung cancer. Those living in high-density areas who are constantly exposed to polluted air are more likely to acquire lung cancer.

The particulate matter in polluted air has been classified as a carcinogen. These small particles get accumulated in the lungs, which may damage DNA in cells and result in cancer. It is strongly advised to concentrate on not smoking, keeping a healthy weight, and cutting alcohol intake if someone wants to lower cancer risks. There must be attempts by the public and the authorities to lower air pollution by choosing healthy and environmentally friendly options, for example, transportation choices like walking, cycling, or driving vehicles with low emissions.

Genetic factors

As you read in the cell division section of the previous chapter, abnormal divisions of cells attributed to dysregulated cell cycles or abnormal genetic changes (mutations) can cause cancer. The genes from parents pass on to their children. So, a family history of lung cancer increases the risk of developing lung cancer significantly. There are findings that indicate that some specific genetic variants are tightly linked with increased chances of lung cancer development in families. Siblings and children of people who have had lung cancer may be at a slightly increased risk of developing the disease themselves, particularly if the relative was diagnosed at a young age. Through research, some specific genetic mutations have been identified that can cause lung cancer.

Previous Lung Disease

Lung cancer risk is higher in people who have a history of chronic lung diseases. Lung cancer is far more likely in patients with Chronic Obstructive Pulmonary Disease (COPD), which comprises disorders including emphysema and chronic bronchitis. Chronic inflammation and lung tissue damage caused by COPD create an environment suitable for cancer development. Research shows that those with COPD are much more likely than those without COPD to develop lung cancer. Likewise, pulmonary fibrosis—which is marked by scar tissue building in the lungs—increases the risk. In pulmonary fibrosis, the scarring process creates an environment whereby aberrant cells can proliferate uncontrollably and cause cancer. Lung cancer is far more likely to affect patients with pulmonary fibrosis than among the general population. Moreover, those who have had lung cancer in the past are more prone to develop it again in the future. A high recurrence risk is also associated with the maintenance of the risk factors that first caused lung cancer, such as cigarette smoking or environmental pollution. Tissue damage and chronic inflammation are the processes driving the higher risk. Chronic inflammation in COPD and pulmonary fibrosis destroys lung tissue and DNA, so aggravating conditions for cancer development.

Infections

There is strong evidence that infections may play a role in the development and progression of lung cancer, suggesting a close relationship between the two. An infection that affects the respiratory system can increase the risk of lung cancer.

The human papillomavirus, also known as HPV is a group of more than 200 viruses. Usually, they do not cause any serious conditions in immunocompetent individuals, but their infection by some high-risk strains can cause diseases of the genitals, for example, genital warts, and cervical cancer. In research, certain viral or genetic strains of the human papillomavirus (HPV) have been discovered to be associated with the development of lung cancer. The potential mechanism involves the ability of these viruses to induce genetic mutations and malignant cellular alterations in the lung tissue, thereby heightening the likelihood of cancer development.

Mycobacterium tuberculosis, the causative agent of tuberculosis (TB), is another major infectious agent. The chronic inflammatory response and tissue damage, e.g., scarring caused by tuberculosis infection, create a favourable environment, which may increase the risk of lung cancer in people with a family history of the disease.

There is multiple ongoing studies to establish a possible link between lung cancer and viral infections, such as EBV (Epstein-Barr virus) and CMV (Cytomegalovirus). Chronic inflammation due to infection by these viruses can suppress immunity and cause cancer development.

A possible connection between Helicobacter pylori and lung cancer is being established, but it is a topic of more research. Helicobacter pylori is a bacterium that resides inside the human gut and is known for its involvement in the development of stomach cancer. But the evidence suggests that it may have an impact on the development of lung cancer as well.

Infections can affect lung cancer in many ways: by impacting the disease's development, its course, and future consequences. Understanding these connections certainly helps health care professionals better develop strategies for the prevention, early detection, and effective treatment of lung cancer.

Chapter 5: Clinical features of Lung Cancer

Lung cancer can manifest through a variety of symptoms, each reflecting different aspects of the disease.

Signs and Symptoms

Chronic Cough:

A chronic cough is one of the first and most common signs of lung cancer. Unlike a typical cough caused by a cold or flu, a cancer-related cough lasts for weeks or even months and does not respond to over-the-counter medications. Coughs can be dry or productive. Coughing usually occurs when a tumour in the lungs causes irritation.

Hemoptysis

Hemoptysis is coughing up blood or blood-tinged sputum. This alarming symptom can range from small blood streaks mixed with mucus to large amounts of blood. It occurs when a lung tumour invades blood vessels in the lungs, resulting in bleeding. Even a small amount of blood in the sputum should prompt an immediate medical evaluation because it can indicate serious underlying conditions, such as lung cancer.

Dyspnea

Dyspnea, or shortness of breath, is a common symptom of lung cancer. It can occur for a variety of reasons, including a tumour obstructing major airways, reducing the amount of air that reaches the lungs; pleural effusion, in which fluid accumulates around the lungs, limiting their expansion; or cancer spreading to lung tissue, reducing lung capacity. Patients may struggle to complete everyday tasks, such as climbing stairs or walking short distances, without feeling breathless.

Wheezing

Wheezing is a high-pitched whistling sound made while exhaling. This symptom can develop when a lung tumour partially obstructs the airways, forcing air through a narrowed passage. While wheezing is commonly associated with asthma and other airway-related respiratory conditions, it can be present in lung cancer due to obstruction or compression of the airways.

Chest pain

Chest pain from lung cancer can vary in nature and intensity. It could be sharp, dull, constant, or intermittent. The pain usually worsens with deep breathing, coughing, or laughing and can spread to the shoulders, or the back. This condition worsens when a tumour invades the chest wall, pleura, or ribs.

Hoarseness of voice

Prolonged hoarseness or changes in voice quality may be another symptom in lung cancer. This symptom occurs when a lung tumour compresses the recurrent laryngeal nerve, which regulates the movement of the vocal cords for producing sound. The pressure damages the nerve, resulting in a hoarse voice.

Recurrent respiratory infections

Recurrent respiratory infections, such as bronchitis or pneumonia, that are difficult to treat or persist, may indicate lung cancer. Tumours can block the airways, allowing bacteria and viruses to grow and cause recurrent infections. These infections may be treated temporarily with antibiotics, but they frequently recur, indicating an underlying obstruction caused by a tumour.

Other systemic symptoms

Weight loss

Cancer cells consume energy, leading to increased metabolic demands and unexplained weight loss. In addition, the body may release substances such as cytokines, which can increase inflammation and alter metabolism. This interference decreases appetite and contributes to weight loss.

Fatigue

Persistent fatigue is a common symptom of lung cancer that does not improve with rest. This extreme tiredness can be caused by the body's efforts to fight the cancer, cancer treatment side effects, anemia (low red blood cell count), or metabolic changes caused by the cancer.

Loss of appetite

Lung cancer can cause appetite loss, resulting in weight loss and malnutrition. This loss of appetite can be caused by the tumour's physical effects, such as pain or difficulty swallowing, or by the cancer's systemic effects, such as metabolic changes and the production of inflammatory cytokines that influence hunger.

Bone Pain:

When lung cancer spreads to the bones, it can cause severe pain. This pain is often constant and can be worse at night or during physical activity. Bone metastases can also lead to fractures, as the cancer weakens the bone structure.

Neurological Symptoms:

If lung cancer spreads to the brain, it can cause a variety of neurological symptoms. These include persistent headaches, seizures, weakness or numbness in the limbs, dizziness, balance problems, and cognitive changes such as confusion or disorientation.

Liver Symptoms:

When lung cancer metastasizes to the liver, it can cause symptoms such as jaundice (yellowing of the skin and eyes), abdominal pain or swelling, and nausea. Liver metastases can also lead to elevated liver enzymes detected through blood tests.

Lymph Node Enlargement:

In cases of lung cancer, swollen lymph nodes, particularly in the neck or above the collarbone, can indicate the spread of lung cancer. These lymph nodes may be palpable and painful. Lymph node involvement is a common pathway for cancer metastasis and often signifies an advanced stage of the disease.

Paraneoplastic Syndromes

Paraneoplastic syndrome is a group of rare disorders that occur when cancer causes symptoms in parts of the body not directly affected by the tumour. These symptoms are caused by the immune system's response to the cancer or by substances released by the cancer cells.

Hypercalcemia:

Some lung cancers, particularly squamous cell carcinoma, can produce parathyroid hormone-related protein (PTHrP), which leads to elevated levels of calcium in the blood. The increased levels of calcium in the blood are called hypercalcemia and associated symptoms with it may include nausea, vomiting, constipation, abdominal pain, excessive thirst, frequent urination, muscle weakness, confusion, etc.

SIADH (Syndrome of Inappropriate Antidiuretic Hormone Secretion):

Small Cell Lung Cancer (SCLC) can produce antidiuretic hormone (ADH), leading to SIADH. This condition causes the body to retain water and dilute the blood sodium levels, leading to hyponatremia (low sodium levels). Symptoms of hyponatremia include fatigue, nausea, headache, muscle cramps, irritability, and, in severe cases, seizures and coma.

Cushing's Syndrome:

Some lung cancers, particularly SCLC, can produce adrenocorticotropic hormone (ACTH), leading to increased levels of cortisol in the blood. Symptoms of Cushing's syndrome include weight gain (particularly around the abdomen and face), high blood pressure, high blood sugar levels, muscle weakness, and skin changes.

Neurological Syndromes:

Lung cancer can cause paraneoplastic neurological syndromes, which are rare disorders triggered by the immune system's response to the cancer. Examples include Lambert-Eaton myasthenic syndrome, characterized by muscle weakness and fatigue, and paraneoplastic cerebellar degeneration, causing problems with coordination, balance, and speech.

Chapter 6: Diagnosis

Diagnosing lung cancer poses a big challenge in its treatment process. It requires the collaboration of experts such as pulmonologists, pathologists, radiologists, surgeons and microbiologists to arrive at an accurate diagnosis. The initial phase of diagnosis entails an examination of the patients' background, identification of pertinent symptoms and signs and a comprehensive physical assessment conducted by a physician. These initial steps play a role in establishing an evaluation that directs subsequent diagnostic procedures and treatment plans.

It involves multiple steps and specialties, for example, pulmonologists, pathologists, radiologists, surgeons, microbiologists, etc., in making the correct diagnosis. The initial steps in diagnosing involve a detailed review of the patient's clinical history, identification of relevant symptoms and signs, and a comprehensive physical examination by a physician. These steps are crucial in forming a preliminary assessment that guides further diagnostic testing and management.

Medical History

Recording a medical history by the doctor involves asking questions about the symptoms (present illness), past history (past illness), co-morbidities, personal history, family history, lifestyle, occupational history, etc.

Symptom Assessment

The primary focus during the medical history assessment revolves around understanding the symptoms experienced by patients with lung cancer. Reported symptoms include-

- **Coughing:** Persistent coughing that may be chronic or acute in onset and productive or non-productive in nature. It might also be accompanied by coughing up blood (Hemoptysis).

- **Loss of appetite and weight Loss:** notable weight loss is often observed as a symptom, among individuals battling cancer.

- **Shortness of Breath:** A gradual development of breathing difficulties (dyspnea) is another symptom frequently encountered in cases of lung cancer. There may be several reasons for these symptoms to develop. This could be due to a blockage in the airway (airway obstruction) or fluid accumulation around the lungs (pleural effusion).

- **Other Symptoms:** These can include chest pain, fatigue, hoarseness, recurrent infections (like pneumonia or bronchitis), and wheezing.

Assessment of Risk Factors: The doctor will inquire about lifestyle factors and risk exposures:

- **Smoking History:** Smoking is the most significant risk factor for lung cancer. Tobacco use is the risk factor for lung cancer. The healthcare provider will ask about how long and how much the individual has smoked (number of cigarettes per day) and whether they currently smoke or have quit.

- **Exposure to Carcinogens:** Occupational and environmental contact with cancer causing substances (carcinogens), like asbestos radon and certain chemicals.

- **Family History:** A family history of lung cancer or other cancers is always asked and recorded as it can indicate a strong genetic predisposition.

Physical Examination

The physical examination is about examining and recording clinical signs that helps identify any underlying conditions.

General Physical Examination: Key components include:

- **Vital signs:** Measurement of weight, height, body mass index (BMI), body temperature, respiratory rate, blood pressure (BP), pulse rate, etc.

- **General Inspection:** Examination of the eyes, hands, feet, and skin for signs such as pallor (pale appearance of the eyes, skin, and nail beds), icterus (yellowish pigmentation of the skin caused by the deposition of bile pigments), cyanosis (bluish discoloration indicating low oxygen levels), clubbing (a condition where the fingertips become bulbous and may indicate chronic hypoxia), pedal edema, examination of lymph nodes to assess lymphadenopathy (enlargement of lymph node) etc.

- The doctor may palpate the lymph nodes in the neck (cervical lymph nodes) and armpits (axillary lymph nodes) for enlargement or tenderness, which may suggest metastasis.

After completing the history-taking and general examination, based on their observations and findings, doctors typically further proceed to examine specific systems, for example, respiratory, cardiovascular, neurological, etc.

Respiratory System Examination: If history, symptoms and signs suggest thoracic involvement, a more detailed examination of upper airway and the chest is performed using:

- **Inspection:** The doctor looks for asymmetry, chest wall deformities, or any visible changes over skin.

- **Palpation:** Feeling the chest wall to detect tenderness, lumps, or abnormal movement during respiration.

- **Percussion:** Tapping on the chest wall to assess the underlying lung structure. A dull sound may indicate fluid, consolidation, or mass.

- **Auscultation:** Listening to the lung sounds using a stethoscope. Abnormal sounds such as wheezing, crackles, or absence of breath sounds suggest underlying pathology like tumours, obstructive processes, pleural effusions, etc.

Importance of the Physical Examination in Diagnosis in Lung Cancer:

A thorough physical examination can reveal signs that are critical for early detection and localization of lung cancer:

- **Clubbing:** Clubbing of the fingers may indicate long-standing hypoxia, which can be associated with chronic lung conditions, including cancer.

- **Enlarged Lymph Nodes:** Swollen lymph nodes can indicate metastasis.

- **Respiratory Signs:** Abnormal respiratory sounds or findings on percussion can prompt further imaging studies to identify lung masses, effusions, or other abnormalities.

Guiding Further Investigations

Following an examination, it is recommended to conduct tests to confirm the findings.

Imaging Procedures: If any irregularities are observed during the examination, additional imaging tests, like chest X-rays, CT scans, or PET scans, may be needed to get a view of the lungs and identify any potentially concerning masses or lesions.

Advance interventions: These include bronchoscopy, thoracoscopy, endobronchial ultrasound, mediastinoscopy, etc. We will learn about these interventions in the upcoming sections. These interventions can be classified as diagnostic and therapeutic procedures. Diagnostic procedures define reaching the underlying pathology to collect samples (tissue or fluid) for diagnostic tests, while therapeutic procedures help remove the underlying pathology to cure the disease or procedures to relieve symptoms.

Biopsy:

In cases where a mass or nodule is detected through imaging or examination, a biopsy is often required. This involves collecting tissue samples from the area for histopathological and molecular analysis, aiding in confirming the diagnosis, determining the specific type of lung cancer, and guiding personalised treatment plans.

Role of Imaging in Lung Cancer Diagnosis

Imaging plays a role in diagnosing, staging, and managing lung cancer. Different imaging techniques are used to visualize the lungs and nearby structures, detect lesions, and assist in diagnostic and treatment decisions. Here are some key types of imaging methods used for diagnosing lung cancer and their respective functions.

Chest X Ray is typically the imaging test conducted when there are suspicions of lung cancer. It offers a cost-effective way to assess the lungs as well as cardiac, soft tissue, and bony structures in the chest area. Chest X rays can identify tumours, collapsed lungs (atelectasis), fluid around the lungs (effusion), and many other irregularities. Despite their advantages, they do have some limitations in spotting very small lesions or those hidden by structures.

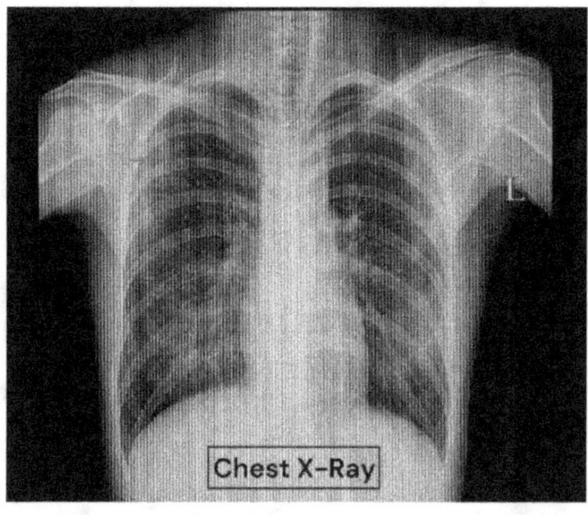

A Computed Tomography (CT) Scan produces sectional images of the body from various angles offering a more thorough view of the lungs compared to chest X rays. Unlike chest X-rays, CT scans excel at detecting small lesions, which is crucial for early lung cancer diagnosis and staging. The detailed CT descriptions help determine tumour size, shape, precise location and involvement of surrounding structures. They also indicate if malignant tissue has spread to lymph nodes or other organs. With CT scan guidance precise diagnostic and therapeutic procedures like needle biopsies on suspected areas can be carried out.

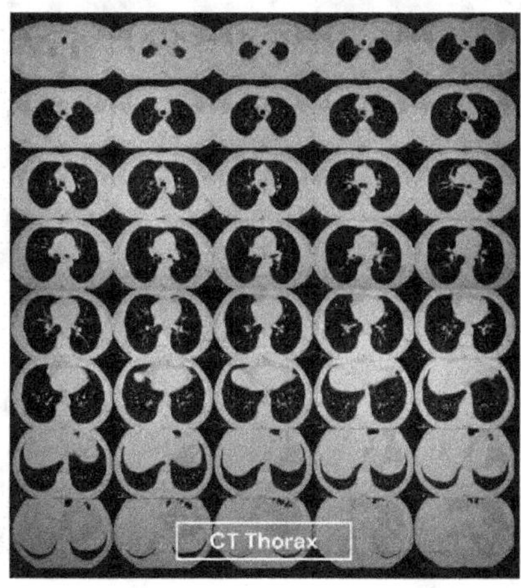

A Positron Emission Tomography (PET) Scan measures metabolic activity and distinguishes between malignant and benign lesions based on glucose uptake levels – cancer cells typically exhibit higher metabolic rates and more glucose uptake. PET scans are valuable for lung cancer staging and pinpointing metastases, offering a picture of disease progression. They also assess the effectiveness of treatment by comparing metabolic activity after therapy. The PET CT scan is an imaging technique that merges features of both CT and PET scans to enhance its sensitivity and accuracy in identifying lung cancer.

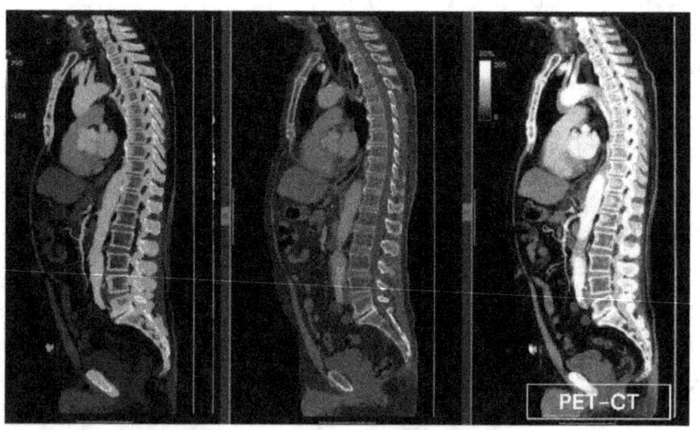

Magnetic Resonance Imaging (MRI) proves valuable in evaluating soft tissue structures and the central nervous system. While not commonly used for lung cancer diagnosis, MRI is vital for detecting brain metastases and providing images of the brain and spinal cord.

Ultrasound is not typically employed for lung cancer diagnosis. It plays a crucial role in guiding procedures like thoracentesis (removal of pleural fluid) and biopsy of peripheral lung lesions. Moreover, ultrasound aids in identifying and assessing effusions or pneumothorax, assisting in the placement of drainage catheters.

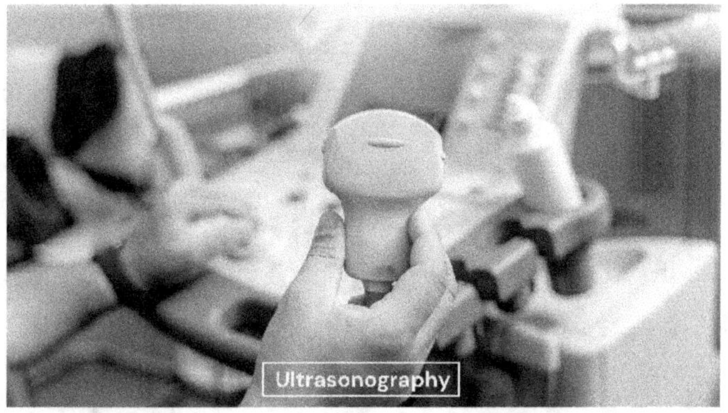

The Radionuclide Bone Scan is utilized to identify the spread of lung cancer to the bones. This imaging method includes injecting an amount of radioactive material and capturing images to highlight regions with abnormal bone metabolism, indicating metastasis. It plays a role in staging and determining the extent of metastatic disease.

The selection of imaging methods often involves an approach beginning with a chest X ray and advancing to detailed imaging techniques such, as CT and PET scans based on initial observations. The combination of imaging methods offers an insight into the illness, aiding in confirming the diagnosis, determining the stage, and devising an appropriate treatment plan. Typically, a diverse team that includes radiologists, oncologists, pulmonologists, and thoracic surgeons evaluates imaging findings to create a treatment strategy. Precise interpretation of imaging results is crucial, for guiding biopsy procedures, planning surgeries, radiation therapy, and others, and evaluating responses to chemotherapy or immunotherapy.

Advanced interventions

Bronchoscopy

Bronchoscopy is an invasive procedure that allows the physician to directly visualize the upper and lower airways, including the nasal cavity, pharynx, larynx, trachea, and bronchial tubes. It is a very effective and commonly used procedure in visualizing tumours, blockages, vocal cord abnormalities, and mucosal abnormalities within the airways. The bronchoscope has many channels within it, which are used for performing several procedures under real-time visualization. These procedures include performing biopsies, bronchoalveolar lavage, etc. from suspicious areas to be analyzed for cancer cells for making the right diagnosis.

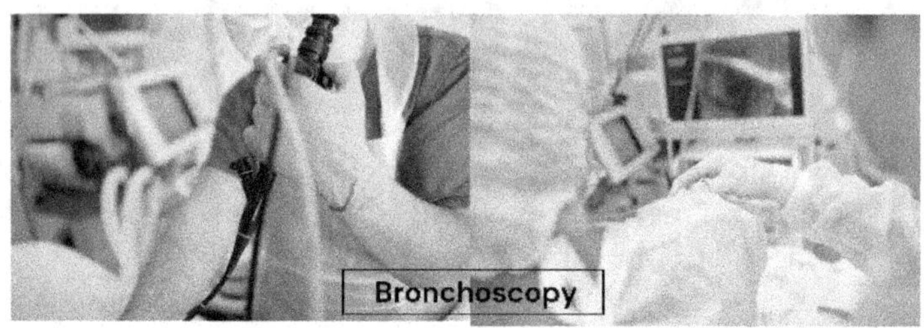

Electromagnetic Navigation Bronchoscopy (EMN):

EMN bronchoscopy is a more advanced technique compared to conventional bronchoscopy. It uses a pre-procedural CT scan of the chest to create a three-dimensional virtual map of the airways. This map guides the doctor to navigate the bronchoscope precisely in order to reach the most peripheral lung areas that are typically not possible to reach with standard bronchoscopy. This enhances the ability to take biopsies from tumours located in the far reaches of the lung, improving diagnostic accuracy for peripheral lung lesions.

Endobronchial Ultrasound (EBUS)

Endobronchial ultrasound (EBUS) is a technique that uses an ultrasound probe at the end of a bronchoscope to view structures in and around the airways, including lymph nodes and blood vessels beyond the airway walls. The EBUS scope provides real-time imaging of the lymph nodes, which enables the physician to guide a needle into the lymph nodes to take tissue samples (transbronchial needle aspiration) for biopsy. EBUS is crucial for staging lung cancer and evaluating the extent of disease spread.

Endoscopic Ultrasound of the Esophagus (EUS)

Esophageal endoscopic ultrasound (EUS) involves inserting an ultrasound probe into the esophagus of the airway allowing for visualization and biopsy of lymph nodes. Both EBUS and EUS play roles in evaluating lymph nodes determining lung cancer stage and guiding treatment plans.

Mediastinoscopy and Mediastinotomy

The mediastinum is a space in the chest between the lungs that houses structures like the heart, blood vessels and lymph nodes. Mediastinoscopy and mediastinotomy differ based on where and how incisions are made. In mediastinoscopy a tube (mediastinoscope) is inserted through an incision above the breastbone to sample lymph nodes, near the trachea and major bronchial areas.

Mediastinoscopy is often performed to take samples from lymph nodes to determine the stage of lung cancer. Mediastinotomy, also called the Chamberlain procedure involves making a cut beside the breastbone to access the mediastinum directly. This method is used when specific lymph nodes cannot be reached through mediastinoscopy.

Thoracoscopy

Thoracoscopy, also known as pleuroscopy, is a major procedure used to investigate the spread of lung cancer to the lungs, chest wall linings, and pleural spaces. During thoracoscopy, a thin tube with a camera (thoracoscope) is inserted through small incisions in the chest wall. The thoracoscope allows direct visualization of the lungs and the pleura around them. The thoracoscope contains many channels through which sampling of tumours, lung tissue, and pleural surfaces can easily be done for further evaluation and investigations.

When combined with video assistance this method is referred to as video assisted surgery (VATS). VATS serves not only for diagnosis but for treatment purposes also. In early-stage lung cancers VATS allows surgeons to remove affected lung parts with the least invasiveness compared to traditional open surgery. This approach offers advantages such as reduced pain, shorter hospital stays and quicker recovery times, for patients.

Summary

Each of these diagnostic procedures plays a crucial role in the diagnosis and management of lung cancer. These techniques provide critical information that helps in making a diagnosis, deciding the stage of the cancer, and guiding treatment decisions. The integration of advanced technologies like electromagnetic navigation and ultrasound-guided biopsies enhances the precision and efficacy of lung cancer diagnostics and interventions, ultimately contributing to improved prognosis and survival rates.

Role of Biopsy in Diagnosing Lung Cancer

Biopsies are crucial for diagnosing lung cancer as they allow experts to closely examine tissue samples providing evidence. The choice of biopsy technique is influenced by the patients' health, the lesions accessibility and the suspected tumour's location. There are different types of biopsies used in lung cancer diagnosis.

1. Needle Biopsy

- Fine Needle Aspiration (FNA): This method involves using a needle to extract tissue or fluid samples from the lung or nearby lymph nodes.
- Core Needle Biopsy: A larger needle is used to obtain a core tissue sample for more in-depth analysis.

Needle biopsies can be guided by ultrasound, CT, or Fluoroscopy to target the lesion site. They are minimally invasive and particularly effective for examining lymph nodes and peripheral lung lesions that bronchoscopy may not reach.

2. Bronchoscopy guided Biopsy

Endobronchial Biopsy: This procedure focuses on obtaining tissue samples from the lining of the bronchial airways specifically targeting lesions or abnormalities, within or closely connected to the walls. This method is commonly used to identify tumours, infections or other irregularities within the tubes. It is highly effective in diagnosing endobronchial growths or lesions.

Transbronchial biopsy: This procedure involves taking tissue samples from lung tissue beyond the bronchial tube walls. The bronchoscope is guided into the tubes to reach the lung regions and a transbronchial biopsy forceps, which pierces the bronchial walls, is used to take the samples. This technique is utilized for diagnosing conditions affecting lung parenchyma such as lung diseases, pulmonary fibrosis, infections or diffuse lung issues.

Transbronchial Needle Aspiration (TBNA): In TBNA a needle is inserted through the wall to extract tissue or lymph node samples near the airways. TBNA is particularly useful for sampling mediastinal lymph nodes or tumours adjacent to the bronchial airways. It is frequently used in staging lung cancer, diagnosing sarcoidosis and assessing conditions affecting lymph nodes or tissues around the airways. Despite being minimally invasive TBNA can provide insights. Each of these methods, endobronchial biopsy, transbronchial biopsy and transbronchial needle aspiration uses a bronchoscope with distinct areas of focus and diagnostic goals.

3. Endoscopic Ultrasound-Guided Biopsy

Types:

Endobronchial Ultrasound Guided Transbronchial Needle Aspiration (EBUS TBNA): Employing a bronchoscope with an ultrasound probe to visualize and sample lymph nodes and masses within or near the airways.

Endoscopic Ultrasound Guided Fine Needle Aspiration (EUS FNA): Inserting an endoscope with an ultrasound probe into the esophagus to sample lymph nodes or masses in proximity to the esophagus.

These advanced techniques enable sampling of lymph nodes and mediastinal structures that may be challenging to access through other means. EBUS TBNA and EUS FNA are particularly useful for staging lung cancer by determining if cancer has spread to the lymph nodes, which's vital for treatment planning

4. Surgical Biopsy

Types:

Mediastinoscopy involves putting an incision above the sternum to insert a mediastinoscope for sampling lymph nodes in the mediastinum.

Mediastinotomy; Requires an incision to provide direct access, to mediastinal structures beyond reach by mediastinoscopy.

Thoracoscopy (Video Assisted Thoracoscopic Surgery. VATS):

Inserting a thoracoscope through incisions in the chest is used to view and take samples of lung tissue or pleural lesions.

Open Lung Biopsy: A procedure involving a larger chest incision is performed to directly access and sample lung tissue.

Surgical biopsies are typically done when other less invasive methods don't give definite results or when a larger tissue sample is needed. Mediastinoscopy and mediastinotomy are commonly used to obtain tissue samples from lymph nodes of the mediastinum, while thoracoscopy (VATS) can be used to examine and take samples from both lung and pleural lesions. Although open lung biopsy is an invasive and surgical procedure, it provides extensive tissue samples crucial for challenging cases where other procedures fail to give a definitive diagnosis.

Non-Invasive Diagnostic Tool

Sputum Cytology

Sputum cytology involves analyzing lung secretions for cells for detecting lung cancer. This method is particularly useful for identifying high risk individuals like smokers and diagnosing central airway malignancies. Despite its lower sensitivity and potential to miss tumours, sputum cytology has some advantages such as easy collection process and minimal discomfort to patients. It is commonly used along with methods to create a comprehensive approach aiding in the early detection of illnesses guiding further testing decisions and monitoring disease progression or treatment response.

Histopathological and Molecular Analysis

The entire process, starting from performing a biopsy to devising a treatment plan requires investigations by pathologists. This critical process not only confirms the presence of cells but also determines their exact type and origin, all essential for tailoring personalized treatments.

Histopathological Analysis

Samples from biopsies or other tissues are sent to a pathology lab where a pathologist studies the cells under a microscope.

- **Microscopic Examination**: The pathologist inspects the tissue to identify cells and determines the type of lung cancer, like non-small cell lung cancer (NSCLC) or small cell lung cancer (SCLC).
- **Special Stains**: Various stains and immunohistochemical methods can be utilized to highlight more specialized components aiding in more precise tumour categorization. Differentiating Between

Differentiation from Metastases:

When examining lung tumours pathologists can distinguish between those that originate within the lungs and those that have spread to the lungs from elsewhere. Identifying the site of the cancer is crucial as treatment approaches vary based on the tumour's origin.

A pathology report is created by synthesizing information gathered from procedures like biopsy, endobronchial biopsy or transbronchial needle aspiration (TBNA). Typically, available for review within a week, this report contains details for diagnosing the patient and devising treatment plans. It not only confirms the presence of cancer and specifies its type, but also provides detailed insights into features like grade, margins and how extensively it impacts surrounding tissues. Based on these findings the pathology report offers recommendations that guide further therapies and management strategies. This comprehensive analysis plays a role in developing a personalized plan of action.

Molecular Analysis of Lung Tumours

Performing molecular or genomic testing on lung tumour samples allows for the identification of specific genetic abnormalities that can potentially impact therapy selection, hence highlighting the importance of tailoring treatment regimens to individual patients. Utilizing sophisticated testing, oncologists can customize treatments based on the genetic characteristics of individual tumours, thereby optimizing the efficacy of targeted therapies and optimizing patient outcomes.

- **Analysis of Genetic Mutations:** KRAS Mutation: Detected in around 20%-25% of patients with non-small cell lung cancer (NSCLC), KRAS mutations have been observed to impact cellular proliferation and viability. Detecting this mutation can help determine the appropriate application of targeted medicines that block the subsequent impacts of KRAS signaling pathways.

- **EGFR Mutation:** Found in 10%-20% of NSCLC cases, EGFR mutations impact the epidermal growth factor receptor, a vital component in cell proliferation and survival. Specific medicines, such as tyrosine kinase inhibitors, can be used to target these mutations.

- **Additional genetic markers:** Additionally, testing for additional significant genes such as ALK, ROS1, RET, BRAF, MET, HER2, and NTRK, among others, is conducted. Each of these genes may have mutations or rearrangements that can be targeted by specialized medicines. ALK and ROS1 rearrangements can be specifically addressed by ALK inhibitors, whereas BRAF mutations can be specifically addressed by BRAF inhibitors. These targeted therapies have shown significant efficacy in patients with corresponding genetic alterations, making genetic marker testing a cornerstone of personalized cancer therapy.

Liquid Biopsy: Liquid biopsy refers to a wide range of minimally invasive procedures that are performed on blood or other physiological fluids to identify fragments of DNA generated from tumours, as well as extracellular vesicles (EVs) and circulating tumour cells (CTCs). The utilization of this sophisticated diagnostic approach has demonstrated substantial promise in the timely identification and treatment of many types of malignancies, such as lung cancer.

- **Circulating tumour DNA (ctDNA):** The primary technique utilised in liquid biopsy for lung cancer is the examination of circulating tumour DNA (ctDNA). This approach is crucial in the initial profiling of genotypes, aiding in the identification of specific genetic alterations within the tumour. Furthermore, ctDNA is highly useful in identifying the mechanisms by which cancer cells develop resistance to targeted medicines, which occurs as a result of mutations and adaptations over time.

In addition to these uses, ctDNA is also employed to assess the efficacy of treatment in individuals receiving therapy. Clinicians can assess the efficacy of the therapy by examining ctDNA levels prior to, during, and post-treatment. In addition, ctDNA has the ability to identify minor residual illness after surgery, which indicates the presence of any remaining cancer cells in the body that may potentially cause a recurrence.

Integration of Pathology and Molecular Testing

The combination of pathological examination and molecular testing forms the backbone of lung cancer diagnosis and treatment planning. By understanding both the tumour's microscopic characteristics and its genetic alterations, clinicians can devise more effective, individualized treatment strategies.

Chapter 7: Lung Cancer Staging

Lung cancer staging is a process that determines the extent of cancer spread within the body. Accurate staging is essential for guiding treatment decisions, predicting prognosis. The most commonly used staging system for lung cancer is the TNM classification, which assesses three key components: the tumour (T), lymph nodes involvement (N), and distant metastasis (M).

TNM Classification System

Primary Tumour (T): The "T" component describes the size and extent of the primary tumour.

- Tis (Carcinoma in Situ): Tumour cells are present but have not invaded deeper tissues.
- T1: Tumour is 3 cm or smaller, surrounded by lung or visceral pleura, and does not invade more proximal bronchus.
    - T1a: Tumour 1 cm or smaller.
    - T1b: Tumour larger than 1 cm but 2 cm or smaller.
    - T1c: Tumour larger than 2 cm but 3 cm or smaller.
- T2: Tumour larger than 3 cm but 5 cm or smaller or has certain features such as invading the visceral pleura, Invading the mainstem bronchus but not involving the carina, or causing atelectasis or obstructive pneumonitis extending to the hilum.
    - T2a: Tumour larger than 3 cm but 4 cm or smaller.
    - T2b: Tumour larger than 4 cm but 5 cm or smaller.
- T3: Tumour larger than 5 cm but 7 cm or smaller, or tumour of any size with direct invasion of chest wall, phrenic nerve, mediastinal or parietal pleural,

parietal pericardium or with satellite tumour nodules within same lobe

- T4: Tumour larger than 7 cm, or tumour of any size Invade any of the following: mediastinum, trachea, recurrent laryngeal nerve, carina, vertebral body, diaphragm, great vessels, or esophagus or satellite tumour nodule within a different lobe of the ipsilateral lung

Regional Lymph Nodes (N): The "N" component describes the involvement of regional lymph nodes:

- NX: Regional lymph nodes cannot be assessed.
- N0: No regional lymph node involvement.
- N1: Metastasis to ipsilateral peribronchial or hilar lymph nodes and intrapulmonary nodes.
- N2: Metastasis to ipsilateral mediastinal and/or subcarinal lymph nodes.
- N3: Metastasis to contralateral mediastinal, contralateral hilar, ipsilateral or contralateral scalene, or supraclavicular lymph nodes.

Distant Metastasis (M): The "M" component describes the presence of distant metastasis:

- M0: No distant metastasis.
- M1: Distant metastasis is present.
    - M1a: Separate tumour nodule(s) in a contralateral lobe, tumour with pleural or pericardial nodules, or malignant pleural or pericardial effusion.
    - M1b: Single extrathoracic metastasis in a single organ.
    - M1c: Multiple extrathoracic metastases in one or more organs.

Understanding the Stages of Lung Cancer

Lung cancer staging helps doctors determine how far cancer has spread within the body, which is essential for choosing the right treatment and understanding the patient's prognosis. Lung cancer is divided into four main stages, from I to IV, with Stage I being the earliest and Stage IV the most advanced.

- Stage I: Early-Stage Lung Cancer: Cancer is found only in the lungs and has not spread to any lymph nodes or other parts of the body. The tumour is relatively small, typically less than 5 centimeters (about 2 inches).
    - Stage IA: The tumour is 3 centimeters (about 1.2 inches) or smaller.
    - Stage IB: The tumour is larger than 3 centimeters but 5 centimeters or smaller.
- Stage II: Localized Lung Cancer: Cancer is still within the lungs but may have spread to nearby lymph nodes or structures within the lung. Tumours can vary in size, but they are still confined to the lungs and nearby areas.
    - Stage IIA: The tumour is larger than 5 centimeters but does not involve nearby lymph nodes.
    - Stage IIB: The tumour may be smaller but has spread to nearby lymph nodes, or it may be larger and involve other parts of the lung or chest wall.
- Stage III: Locally Advanced Lung Cancer: Cancer has spread to nearby lymph nodes and may have invaded other structures within the chest, such as the chest wall, diaphragm, or nearby organs. While it is more extensive than Stage II, it has not yet spread to distant parts of the body.
    - Stage IIIA: Cancer is found in lymph nodes on the same side of the chest as the primary tumour.

- o Stage IIIB: Cancer has spread to lymph nodes on the opposite side of the chest or above the collarbone.
  - o Stage IIIC: Cancer has invaded nearby structures and lymph nodes extensively.
- Stage IV: Advanced or Metastatic Lung Cancer: Cancer has spread beyond the lungs to other parts of the body, such as the liver, bones, brain, or other distant organs. This is the most advanced stage, indicating widespread metastasis.
  - o Stage IVA: Cancer has spread within the chest to other parts of the lung or pleura or to a single distant organ.
  - o Stage IVB: Cancer has spread to multiple distant organs.

Staging of Small Cell Lung Cancer (SCLC)

Small cell lung cancer (SCLC) is an aggressive form of lung cancer characterized by rapid growth and early spread to distant sites. Accurate staging is crucial for determining the appropriate treatment and predicting patient outcomes. Although TNM staging is also applied to SCLC, many clinicians favour another classification system for it. The SCLC can be classified into two stages: limited stage (LS) and extensive stage (ES).

Limited-stage small cell lung cancer (SCLC) is used to describe cancer that is restricted to one side of the chest and can be treated with a single radiation port. This usually involves patients who have lymphadenopathy in the hilar, mediastinal, and ipsilateral (same side) supraclavicular regions.

Extensive stage small cell lung cancer (SCLC) is characterised by the progression of the illness beyond the boundaries of one half of the chest cavity. This encompasses the spread of cancer cells to remote organs, the contralateral lung, or distant lymph nodes. If malignant cells are found in the fluid surrounding the lungs (pleural effusion), this indicates that the disease is in an advanced stage.

A less prevalent stage, referred to as **very limited stage (VLS)**, has been suggested for patients who have small primary tumours and no detectable regional lymphadenopathy or distant metastases.

Understanding the stages of lung cancer helps patients and their families grasp the severity of the disease and the treatment options available. Early detection and treatment significantly improve the chances of successful outcomes.

Chapter 8: Screening for Lung Cancer

Lung cancer is one of the main contributors to global mortality from cancer. Timely identification with the help of screening gives an opportunity to intervene early which eventually enhances the effectiveness of medical interventions and the likelihood of patient survival. This chapter discusses the significance of lung cancer screening, the steps involved, eligibility criteria for screening, and the advantages and disadvantages associated with screening. Early detection of lung cancer significantly enhances the potential for effective management through interventions such as surgery, radiation, and targeted therapy. The main purpose of screening is to identify lung cancer before the onset of symptoms.

The Screening Procedure

The screening process begins with an initial risk assessment by a healthcare professional to determine if an individual is at high risk for lung cancer. This assessment typically considers factors such as age, smoking history, and exposure to carcinogens.

Eligibility for Lung Cancer Screening

Screening recommendations primarily apply to adults aged 50 to 80 years who have a significant smoking history. The criteria include:

- Adults between 50 and 80 years old.
- Individuals with a 20-pack-year smoking history who currently smoke or have quit within the past 15 years.

A pack year is a way to quantify smoking history. One pack-year is equivalent to smoking one pack of cigarettes per day for one year. For example, a 20-pack-year history could mean smoking one pack a day for 20 years or two packs a day for 10 years.

The screening age range and smoking pack years have recently been updated by the United States Preventive Services Task Force (USPSTF). They updated the guideline to expand the age range for screening from 55–80 years to 50–80 years and to reduce the smoking history requirement from 30 pack-years to 20 pack-years. This update intends to include more individuals at risk who may benefit from early detection.

Low-Dose CT (LDCT) Scan:

Individuals identified as high risk are offered a low dose computed tomography (LDCT) scan. LDCT is as similar as a usual CT scan, except that LDCT uses a lower radiation dose. The low radiation dose is important to minimize the risk associated with radiation exposure.

Those who are at high risk of developing lung cancer are typically advised to have annual LDCT scans to ensure ongoing monitoring and early detection of any new abnormalities.

Benefits and Risks of Lung Cancer Screening

Benefits:

- **Early Detection:** The primary goal of screening is to detect lung cancer at an early, more treatable stage.

- **Increased Survival Rates:** Early-stage lung cancers have a better prognosis, and early treatment can significantly improve survival rates.

- **Monitoring High-Risk Individuals:** Regular screening helps monitor those at high risk, ensuring timely intervention if cancer develops.

Risks:

- **Radiation Exposure:** Although LDCT uses lower radiation doses than conventional CT scans, there is still some exposure to radiation.

- **False Positives/Negatives:** Screening can sometimes yield false-positive results, leading to unnecessary anxiety and additional tests. Conversely, false negatives may miss existing cancers.

- **Overdiagnosis:** Screening may detect cancers that would not have caused symptoms or affected the individual's lifespan, leading to potential overtreatment.

Deciding whether to undergo lung cancer screening is a personal decision that should be based on careful consideration of the potential benefits and risks. Individuals eligible for screening are encouraged to discuss their options with their healthcare providers. Healthcare providers can offer guidance tailored to everyone's situation, helping them make an informed decision.

Chapter 9: Treatment Lung Cancer

Upon receiving a diagnosis, it is crucial to determine the treatment for the patient. The choice of treatment is based on factors such as the type and stage of cancer well as the overall health condition of the individual. This segment provides an overview of the treatment options for lung cancer followed by an explanation of each option.

Treatment Overview

The primary objective of treating lung cancer varies depending on the disease's stage. In cases of early-stage lung cancer the main goal typically aims at achieving a cure. However, as the cancer advances to higher stages the focus shifts towards managing the illness and easing symptoms to enhance the patient's quality of life.

Early-stage lung cancer (Stages I and II): Treatments for early-stage lung cancer, which includes Stages I and II, usually consist of surgical removal of the tumour. After surgery, additional measures such as chemotherapy or radiotherapy may be considered to ensure the total elimination of any lingering cancer cells.

Locally advanced lung cancer (Stage III): For locally advanced lung cancer (Stage III), a more comprehensive treatment approach is typically required. This involves a combination of chemotherapy, radiotherapy, and, in certain situations, surgery.

Advanced lung cancer stage (IV): For stage IV lung cancer, the primary goal of treatment is to effectively control the cancer and address symptoms in order to extend the patient's life and enhance their overall quality of life.

Multidisciplinary approach to treatment

Effective lung cancer treatment requires the collaboration of various medical professionals, each with their own specialized expertise. These include thoracic surgeons, medical oncologists, radiation oncologists, pulmonologists, radiologists, pathologists, and palliative care experts. This team works together to create a customized treatment plan that is specifically designed to meet individual needs.

Surgery

Surgery is the first-choice treatment for non-small cell lung cancer (NSCLC) if the cancer is localized and the patient is healthy enough to undergo the operation. The types of lung cancer surgery include:

- **Lobectomy:** Removal of an entire lobe of the lung, the most common surgery for early-stage lung cancer.

- **Segmentectomy or Wedge Resection:** Removal of a part of a lobe, used for smaller tumours or patients who may not tolerate a lobectomy.

- **Pneumonectomy:** Removal of an entire lung, used for large or centrally located tumours.

Radiation Therapy

Radiation therapy uses high-energy rays to kill cancer cells and is often employed in the following scenarios:

- When surgical removal is not an option.

- In combination with chemotherapy, either before or after surgery.

- To relieve symptoms in advanced cancer stages.

Chemotherapy

Chemotherapy involves the use of drugs to kill cancer cells, administered intravenously or orally. It can be used:

- **Before Surgery (Neoadjuvant Therapy):** To shrink tumours.

- **After Surgery (Adjuvant Therapy):** To kill any remaining cancer cells.

- **As the Main Treatment:** For cancers that have spread.

Targeted Therapy and Immunotherapy

Advances in understanding lung cancer genetics and immune evasion have led to the development of targeted therapies and immunotherapy.

Targeted Therapy: These drugs focus on specific mutations in cancer cells, blocking their growth and spread while minimizing damage to normal cells. Examples include drugs targeting EGFR mutations and ALK rearrangements.

Immunotherapy: Immunotherapy enhances the body's natural defenses to fight cancer, helping the immune system recognize and attack cancer cells. Checkpoint inhibitors like pembrolizumab and nivolumab are examples of immunotherapy agents used in lung cancer treatment.

Lung cancer therapy is multifaceted and dynamic, aiming not only to prolong life but also to control symptoms and maintain or improve quality of life. A comprehensive discussion with the healthcare team ensures that patients understand the benefits and risks of all available options, allowing them to make informed decisions aligned with their values and goals.

Surgery

Surgery is a common lung cancer treatment option that is considered in patients with early-stage NSCLC and in some cases of SCLC cancer. This section focuses on surgical lung cancer treatments, types of surgeries, and what someone can expect during recovery following surgery.

The primary goal of lung cancer surgery is to eliminate all cancerous tissue. Consequently, a section of the diseased lung, or in rare cases, the entire lung, may be removed. Surgery is most successful when the cancer is localized and there have been no distant metastases. There are several surgical techniques that can be applied for lung cancer treatment. The type of surgery is decided based on the patient's overall health, tumour's size and characteristics, as well as the stage of the cancer.

Types of Resection Techniques

1. Lobectomy: Lobectomy is the surgical removal of a whole lung lobe, and it is the preferred procedure for early-stage cancers. Human lungs have five lobes: three on the right and two on the left; therefore, removing the lobe containing the tumour provides the highest chance of curing it. Lobectomy can be performed using either classic open surgery, known as thoracotomy, or minimally invasive procedures i.e. robotic or video-assisted thoracoscopic surgery. (Fig. 9.1)

2. Segmentectomy-Each lobe of the lung has a few segments within it. There are 10 segments in the right lung and 8 in the left lung, each with a different size and blood supply. Segmentectomy, also known as sublobar resection, involves removing only a segment or a portion of a lung lobe. These procedures are used for patients with tiny tumours (<2 cm). (Fig. 9.1)

3. Wedge resection: Wedge resection is the surgical excision of a tiny, wedge-shaped piece of the lung that surrounds the tumour. It is mainly reserved for cases where the patient has contraindications for other forms of excisions due to various morbidities or the inability to execute the procedure due to reduced lung function.

4. Pneumonectomy: Pneumonectomy is one of the most extensive lung tumour removal methods. Pneumonectomy is the removal of a complete lung. This approach is utilised when the tumour is too large for a lobectomy or is centrally positioned enough to affect all main organs. (Fig. 9.1)

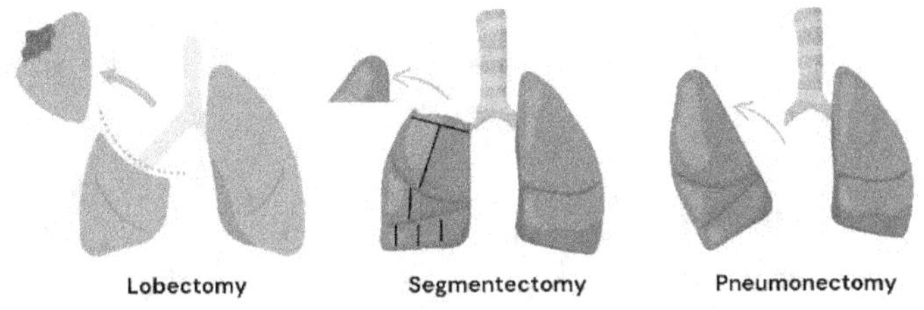

(Fig. 9.1: Illustrating different resection techniques)

Minimally Invasive Surgical Techniques

Minimally invasive thoracic surgery is a surgical technique that involves doing operations using small incisions, without the need for major cuts or spreading of the ribs. Surgeons employ a camera and specialized equipment to gain access to the lungs through these incisions. The two main techniques are video-assisted thoracoscopic surgery (VATS) and robotic-assisted surgery. During VATS, a thoracoscope equipped with a camera is placed through a small incision, enabling the surgeon to observe the chest cavity and remove lung tissue through other small incisions. Robotic-assisted surgery entails the surgeon manipulating robotic equipment and a 3D camera from a console, allowing for accurate extraction of lung tissue through small incisions.

Post-Surgery Recovery

Recovery after surgery varies for each patient, depending on the extent of the surgery and overall health. Key aspects of post-surgery recovery include:

- **Pain Management:** Postoperative pain is common, and its management is essential for better recovery.

Pain medication, nerve blocks, and other analgesic methods can be used.

- **Respiratory Care and Occupational Therapy:** Respiratory and occupational therapists can assist the patient with breathing exercises and provide an incentive spirometer (fig. 9.2), which is used for breathing exercises that help expand the lungs and improve their function.

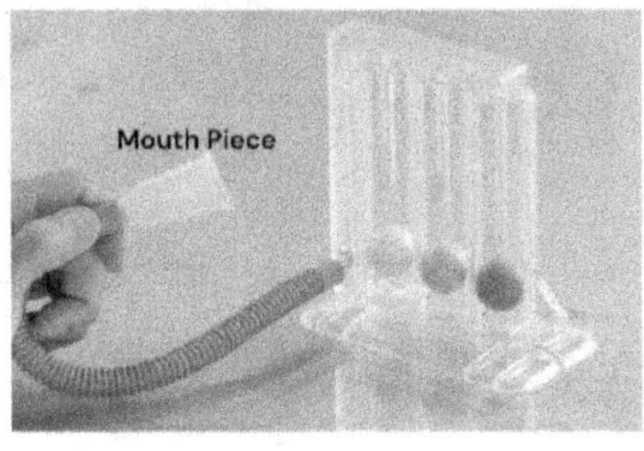

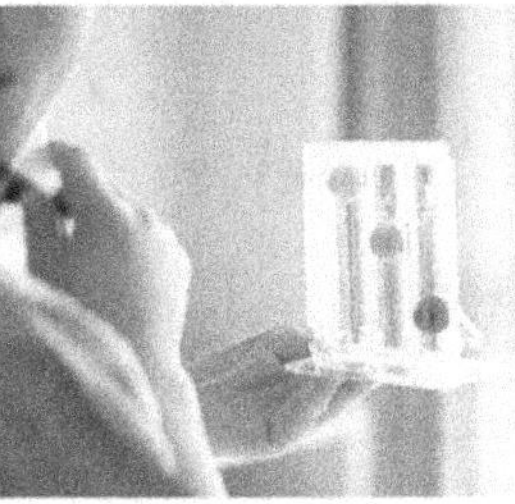

(Fig. 9.2: Incentive Spirometer: Patient is asked to take slow deep breaths through the device's mouthpiece)

- **Early Mobilization:** Patients are advised to engage in early mobilization, including walking, and should progressively increase their activity levels as they recover.

- **Monitoring for Complications:** Complications such as infections, bleeding, and dehiscence of the sutures may arise. Hospital staff and follow-up visits are necessary for monitoring and managing these complications.

- **Long-term Follow-up:** Regular follow-up is required to assess lung function, manage any long-term consequences of surgery, and detect cancer recurrence early.

When caught early enough, lung cancer surgery can increase the likelihood of a cure or significantly extend survival time.

For optimal results, appropriate patient selection, proper postoperative care, and a thorough assessment of the risks and benefits of the procedure are critical.

Radiation Therapy

Radiation therapy, as the name itself suggests, is a therapy that uses high-energy radiation to kill cancer cells. Its applications in management are wide-ranging. It can be used as a primary therapy, as an adjunctive therapy alongside surgery, or as a palliative therapy for symptom control in advanced cancer. This section discusses the intricacies of radiation therapy for lung cancer, including the mechanisms, types, and what patients can expect before, during, and after radiotherapy. The radiotherapy they receive may be thoracic radiotherapy (targeting tumour cells in the lung) or radiotherapy against metastatic sites, for instance, brain or bone metastases.

How Radiation Therapy Works

As you know, mutations in genetic materials (DNA) are the reasons for the development of malignancy. In radiation therapy, the high energy radiation falls on cancer cells and damages their DNAs to the extent that the cells cannot further divide and eventually die. Since the radiation has the potential to affect both cancer and normal cells, extreme care is taken to minimize the damage to the surrounding normal cells. There are several techniques followed for achieving precise targets and calculating the appropriate dose of radiation.

Types of Radiation Therapy

External Beam Radiation Therapy (EBRT)

EBRT is the most common form of radiation therapy for lung cancer. It uses various machines to direct high-energy rays from outside the body into the tumour.

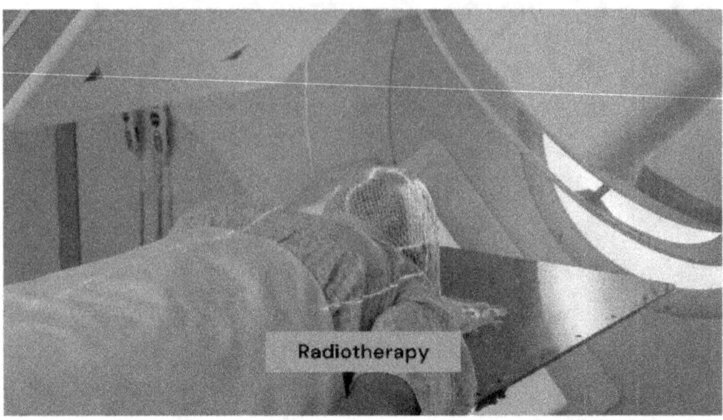

- **Three-Dimensional Conformal Radiation Therapy (3D-CRT):** Utilizes imaging to deliver radiation precisely to the shape of the tumour.

- **Intensity-Modulated Radiation Therapy (IMRT):** Uses advanced technology to modulate the intensity of the radiation beams during therapy and allows more precise targeting of the tumour and sparing normal tissue.

- **Stereotactic Body Radiotherapy (SBRT):** Also known as stereotactic ablative radiotherapy (SABR), SBRT delivers a high dose of radiation in 3 to 5 sessions. It is used mainly for small, early-stage tumours in patients who cannot undergo surgery or for tumours in challenging locations within the lung.

Brachytherapy

Brachytherapy involves placing radioactive material directly close to the cancer cells inside the body, typically through bronchoscopy. It is used less commonly than EBRT or SBRT but can be effective for treating tumours within or near the airways.

What to Expect During Radiation Therapy

Treatment Planning

Before starting radiation therapy, an assessment with CT scans, MRIs, or PET scans is required to determine the precise location of the tumour within the lung. The radiation oncologist uses these images to design a treatment plan that targets the tumour while minimizing exposure to healthy tissues.

During Treatment

Patients typically receive EBRT a few days a week for several weeks, depending on the disease type and extent. Each visit involves setup and positioning, which may take some time, but the actual radiation exposure lasts only a few minutes. The process is painless and similar to getting an X-ray.

Post-Treatment

After completing radiation therapy, patients have follow-up appointments to monitor the response to treatment and manage any late-emerging side effects.

Managing Side Effects

Side effects of radiation therapy depend on the treatment area and radiation dose. Common side effects include:

- **Skin Changes:** Redness, blistering, or peeling in the treated area.

- **Fatigue:** A common and often pervasive side effect.

- **Difficulty Swallowing:** If the radiation area is close to the esophagus, it may become inflamed, causing difficulty swallowing.

- **Pneumonitis:** Inflammation of the lung tissue, usually occurring weeks to months after radiation therapy. Symptoms include coughing and shortness of breath.

- **Radiation Fibrosis:** Long-term scarring of lung tissue, leading to chronic breathing problems.

Managing these side effects is important to maintaining the patient's quality of life. Management strategies may include medications, dietary changes, physical therapy, and supportive care to alleviate symptoms and ensure overall well-being.

Chemotherapy

Chemotherapy, which uses medications known for their capacity to destroy cancer cells, is a crucial strategy in the fight against lung cancer. It is an essential part of the treatment plan for lung cancer patients, regardless of whether their disease is small cell lung cancer (SCLC) or non-small cell lung cancer (NSCLC). Chemotherapy drugs reach the bloodstream either by direct injection or oral ingestion, allowing them to circulate throughout the body and target cancer cells wherever they may be.

Non-Small Cell Lung Cancer (NSCLC)

Chemotherapy is used in non-small-cell lung cancer (NSCLC) for three main purposes: as adjuvant therapy in early-stage disease to prevent recurrence after surgical resection, as concurrent therapy with radiation in locally advanced disease to improve local response and prevent metastasis, and as palliative therapy in advanced disease to ease symptoms and prolong survival.

Types of Chemotherapy

- **Adjuvant chemotherapy** is administered following the primary treatment, such as surgery, with the aim of eradicating any residual cancer cells and minimizing the chances of cancer recurrence. This form of chemotherapy is designed to eliminate microscopic cancer cells that could potentially remain in the body. This leads to enhanced long-term results and increased chances of survival for patients. The standard adjuvant chemotherapy strategy consists of combining platinum-based medications, such as cisplatin or carboplatin, with additional agents, such as paclitaxel, vinorelbine, or gemcitabine. This combination of drugs is known as adjuvant chemotherapy. It has been demonstrated through research that adjuvant chemotherapy has the potential to enhance the five-year survival rate of patients with stage II and IIIA non-small cell lung cancer.

- **Neoadjuvant chemotherapy** involves administering chemotherapy prior to the main treatment, like surgery, for cancer patients. Our objective is to reduce the size of the tumour, facilitating its surgical removal and improving the likelihood of a successful operation. Neoadjuvant chemotherapy is effective in eliminating microscopic cancer cells that might have spread but are still undetectable. As is the case with adjuvant therapy, neoadjuvant chemotherapy frequently involves a regimen that is based on platinum. Neoadjuvant chemotherapy has been shown to improve the long-term survival in patients with stage IIIA non-small cell lung cancer.

- **Concurrent chemoradiotherapy:** The conventional treatment technique for patients with locally advanced non-small cell lung cancer (stage III) is an approach that involves concurrent chemotherapy and radiation therapy. This entails administering radiation therapy and chemotherapy at the same time, which increases the efficiency of both of these treatment techniques. With the help of this combination, the tumour is radiosensitized, which means that cancer cells become more vulnerable to radiation. Both cisplatin and etoposide, as well as carboplatin and paclitaxel, are known to be the most often employed chemotherapeutic drugs in this particular context. In comparison to radiation therapy alone, it has been demonstrated that concurrent chemoradiation is superior in terms of both the local control of the disease and the overall survival rate.

- **In Conjunction with Targeted Therapy and Immunotherapy:** Chemotherapy may be combined with targeted therapies and immunotherapies as well based on the presence of certain specific mutations. The introduction of immunotherapy and targeted medicines has brought about a change in the landscape of non-small cell lung cancer treatment. Drugs like as erlotinib, crizotinib, and osimertinib are able to target certain genetic mutations that have been identified through the process of molecular profiling of tumours. These mutations include EGFR, ALK, and ROS1, among others. In comparison to traditional chemotherapy, these targeted medicines provide a more individualised approach to treatment, which frequently results in fewer adverse effects and better overall therapeutic success. There has also been a revolution in the treatment of advanced non-small cell lung cancer by the use of immunotherapy, specifically immune checkpoint inhibitors such as pembrolizumab and nivolumab. PD-L1 expression patients have demonstrated considerable survival benefits from these medicines, which increase the immune response of the body against cancer cells and have shown significant survival benefits.

- **Palliative chemotherapy:** Palliative chemotherapy is primarily administered to patients with advanced or metastatic non-small cell lung cancer (stage IV) for the purpose of palliative care, which includes the alleviation of symptoms, improvement of quality of life, and extending the duration of survival. As a conventional first-line treatment, platinum-based doublets, such as cisplatin or carboplatin coupled with medicines such as paclitaxel, gemcitabine, pemetrexed, or docetaxel, are utilised. It has been found that pemetrexed is particularly successful in treating non-squamous histologies, whereas other medicines may be more beneficial in treating squamous cell carcinoma. Despite the fact that palliative chemotherapy cannot cure cancer, it has the potential to greatly increase life expectancy and decrease symptoms associated with the disease.

Small Cell Lung Cancer (SCLC)

Chemotherapy for small cell lung cancer (SCLC) can be divided into first-line and second-line regimens. Unlike non-small cell lung cancer (NSCLC), SCLC shows high sensitivity to chemotherapy, likely due to its rapid growth rate. Chemotherapy significantly prolongs survival in SCLC patients, with untreated patients rarely surviving more than a few months. In limited stage (LS) SCLC, combining chemotherapy with thoracic radiation achieves high response rates. In extensive stage (ES) SCLC, chemotherapy does shows some response but the overall median survival still remains low, usually a few months only.

The first treatments for small cell lung cancer (SCLC) consisted of alkylating drugs such as nitrogen mustard and cyclophosphamide. However, the focus quickly switched to medication combinations in order to achieve better results. CAV, which stands for cyclophosphamide, doxorubicin, and vincristine, was a standard first-line therapy up until the middle of the 1980s. Since then, platinum-based regimens have been the standard, notably cisplatin coupled with etoposide, which has demonstrated good efficacy while exhibiting relatively lesser or controlled toxicity. This regimen is normally repeated every three weeks for a total of four to six cycles. Carboplatin is frequently utilised in place of cisplatin because of its more favourable toxicity profile. In the past many years, several other combinations have also been tried, but in general, the most effective first-line treatment for the majority of patients with small cell lung cancer (SCLC) is still etoposide-platinum chemotherapy, with thoracic radiation added wherever required.

- **Addition of Immunotherapeutic Medicines:** Drugs such as atezolizumab or durvalumab are often added to the chemotherapy regimen to enhance the immune response against cancer cells. This combination has shown promising results in extending survival and improving quality of life.

Methods of Administration of Chemotherapy

The administration of chemotherapy medications can be done in a number of different ways, including by intravenous injections and oral administration. The mode of administration is determined by the type of drug, the personalized treatment plan, and sometimes the patient's decision or condition as well.

Intravenous Administration

Intravenous (IV) administration of chemotherapeutic medicines is the most common method. This can be accomplished by:

- **Inserting a Cannula:** Each treatment session requires the insertion of a cannula, a tiny, thin tube, into a vein in the forearm. This allows the medication to be delivered directly into the bloodstream.

- **Long-Term Access Devices:** For patients undergoing continuous treatment, more permanent options include:

  o **Central Lines:** These types of catheters are placed in large veins. The most common veins are the internal jugular vein of the neck and subclavian vein of the chest.

- o **Peripherally Inserted Central Catheters (PIC Lines):** These are also a type of central lines and they are inserted into veins of the arms.

- o **Portacaths:** The port is implanted under the skin, typically on the right side of the chest. It is connected to a catheter which is threaded into a large vein above the right side of the heart.

Oral Chemotherapy

Some chemotherapy medications can be taken orally in the form of pills. The drugs are absorbed into the bloodstream from the stomach. The absorption can be influenced by factors such as whether the medication is taken with food or on an empty stomach. Therefore, it is crucial to follow the healthcare provider's exact instructions when taking these medicines.

Duration of Treatment

Chemotherapy is typically administered in cycles, each consisting of a treatment phase followed by a recovery period to allow the body to recuperate. For instance, a three-week cycle may consist of a week of treatment followed by a two-week break. The number of cycles and their duration depend on the specific treatment plan and the patient's response to the therapy.

Sites of Chemotherapy Administration

Outpatient Clinics

The majority of cancer patients are treated at cancer day clinics that are open to the public. Patients can get their chemotherapy medications administered at these clinics and go home the same day. Because patients may be required to sit for long amounts of time during treatment, it can be good for them to bring something to occupy their time or someone to converse with.

Home Administration

Home administration of some chemotherapy drugs is possible with the use of a portable pump that provides continuous drug delivery or oral administration. This method offers convenience and comfort, allowing patients to maintain a more normal lifestyle during treatment.

Hospitalization

A stay in the hospital might be required for advanced therapies. Patients in this situation typically require hospitalisation for the administration of medications as well as thorough monitoring to address any possible problems or side effects.

Factors Influencing the Choice of Administration Method

The best method for administering chemotherapy depends on several factors, including:

- **Chemotherapy Drugs:** The specific drugs used and their formulations.

- **Cancer Types:** Different types of cancer may respond better to certain administration methods.

- **Treatment Plans:** Individualized treatment plans tailored to the patient's needs.

- **Patient's General Health:** Overall health and ability to tolerate different administration methods.

- **Lifestyle Considerations:** The patient's lifestyle and personal preferences.

Maintaining open communication with the healthcare team during treatment is essential. Patients should feel comfortable discussing any concerns or side effects that arise.

Pre-Treatment Preparation

In order to ensure that the patient is prepared for chemotherapy and to maximise the effectiveness of the treatment, pre-treatment preparation for chemotherapy includes a number of necessary steps. Initially, a thorough medical evaluation is carried out, which includes blood tests, imaging studies, and evaluations of organ function. The purpose of this evaluation is to establish a baseline health state and identify any potential issues that may affect the patient. It is common practice to recommend to patients that they drink enough of water, consume a diet rich in nutrients, and get plenty of rest in the days preceding up to their prescribed treatment.

Pre-chemotherapy consultations with healthcare experts typically include a discussion of the specific chemotherapy regimen, probable side effects, and management measures. In addition, patients could be required to take medications that have been recommended to them in order to prevent nausea or address any potential adverse effects. Providing patients with emotional and psychological assistance, such as counselling or support groups, can assist them in managing the stress and worry that they experience as a result of undergoing chemotherapy. In addition, it is essential to make practical arrangements, such as managing transportation to and from therapy sessions and coordinating assistance at home. The ability of patients to properly manage the treatment process can be improved by addressing these issues, which will allow them to approach chemotherapy with a clear understanding and a supporting framework.

Side Effects of Chemotherapy

Chemotherapy targets cancer cells but it also has the potential to cause damage to normal cells, results in a wide range of negative effects. The degree and nature of these adverse effects can vary widely depending on the type of medicines that are being administered, the dosage, as well as the patient's response to the treatment. This chapter gives an overview of the common side effects of chemotherapy as well as suggestions to manage them.

Common Side Effects

Nausea and Vomiting

Nausea and vomiting are among the most common side effects of chemotherapy. These symptoms can occur shortly after treatment or several days later. Antiemetics medications are often prescribed to help manage these symptoms. Additionally, patients are encouraged to drink adequate amounts of water, eat small and frequent meals, and avoid oily and spicy foods.

Loss of Appetite

Chemotherapy patients often have less appetite and more need for energy to restore the body, which can lead to weight loss. Working with a dietician or other nutritional support can help control these changes. Choosing nutrient-dense foods heavy in calories and protein and eating small, regular meals can help preserve energy levels and body weight.

Fatigue

A common side effect of chemotherapy is fatigue, sometimes characterised as extreme and depressing tiredness. It can affect everyday activities by causing more morbidity and eventually affecting the standard of living. Patients on chemotherapy should try a mix between rest and light physical activity—such as quick walks or mild stretching—to control tiredness. Besides, maintaining a good amount of sleep is very important, along with light physical activities.

Immune System Suppression

Infections are more likely to occur as a result of chemotherapy since it can impair the immune system. A decrease in the number of white blood cells due to chemotherapy is one of the main reasons of this immunosuppression. There are some preventive measures that patients are encouraged to adopt in order to reduce the risk of catching infections.

- Practicing good hand hygiene

- Avoiding crowded places and meeting lots of people

- Keeping up with vaccinations as recommended by their healthcare provider

It is strongly advised to report any signs of illness, such as fever, chills, cough, or sore throat, to the healthcare team promptly.

Blood Coagulation Issues

The coagulation of blood can be disrupted by chemotherapy, which might result in an increased risk of bruising and bleeding. The reason behind this is that there is a decrease in platelets in patients on chemotherapy, which are important for the process of blood clotting. Patients should stay away from engaging in activities that have the potential to get them injured. Use a gentle toothbrush and take precaution when shaving. Any unusual bleeding, such as nosebleeds or blood in the urine or stool, should be reported immediately to the doctor.

Gastrointestinal Problems

It is possible for chemotherapy to cause gastrointestinal problems, such as diarrhoea or constipation, due to its impact on the digestive tract. Make adjustments to your diet, drink enough water, and take any medications that your healthcare team recommends in order to manage these symptoms. Constipation can be alleviated by drinking plenty of fluids, eating foods high in fibre, and staying active.

Temporary Hair Loss

Many chemotherapeutics drugs cause hair loss by affecting cells in the hair follicles. This type of hair loss is usually temporary, and hair typically begins to grow back after treatment ends.

Mouth Sores

Chemotherapy can cause the lining of the mouth to become sore and prone to ulceration. Maintaining good oral hygiene, using mouth rinses prescribed by a healthcare provider, and avoiding irritating foods (such as spicy and acidic) can help manage this side effect.

Managing Side Effects and Risks

Communication with Healthcare Team

It is essential to notify the treatment team of any adverse effects. They can modify dosages or change medications to enhance the patient's comfort and treatment outcomes. Additionally, supportive care measures, such as medications to manage side effects, nutritional support, and physical therapy, can be implemented.

When to Seek Immediate Medical Attention

Patients should seek immediate medical attention if they experience:

- A rise in body temperature above 37.5°C (99.5°F) or below 36°C (96.8°F)

- Symptoms of infection, such as chills, cough, sore throat, or any other signs of illness

- Unusual bleeding or bruising

- Severe or persistent pain

- Difficulty breathing

Due to low immunity, infections during chemotherapy can quickly escalate to life-threatening complications and that's why it is crucial to intervene early to managing these risks.

Practical Tips for Patients and Families

- **Keep a Symptom Diary:** Track any side effects and their severity to discuss with your healthcare team.

- **Stay Hydrated:** Drink plenty of fluids to help manage side effects like nausea, constipation, and fatigue.

- **Plan Rest Periods:** Schedule time to rest and recover and prioritize activities to conserve energy.

- **Eat Well:** Focus on a balanced diet rich in nutrients to support overall health and recovery.

- **Stay Connected:** Maintain communication with friends and family for emotional support and practical assistance.

Targeted Therapy

Targeted therapy represents a sophisticated approach to combating cancer by focusing on specific genes, receptors, or the tissue environment that supports cancer cell growth and survival. Unlike classic chemotherapy or radiation, which broadly attack rapidly dividing cells, targeted therapy aims to block the specific molecular mechanisms and pathways responsible for the division. This precision makes targeted therapy potentially more effective and less harmful. The primary targets, i.e. genetic mutations and alterations in cancer cells are identified through molecular analysis.

The most common genetic mutations in lung cancer are the following:

- **EGFR (Epidermal Growth Factor Receptor):** This receptor is present on specific cells and has the ability to bind to a substance known as epidermal growth factor. Understanding the intricate mechanisms of cell signaling pathways that govern cell division and survival is crucial. In certain cases, mutations in the EGFR gene can lead to an overproduction of epidermal growth factor receptor proteins, which leads to an increased and uncontrolled division of cancer cells. Mutations in the EGFR gene are common in non-small cell lung cancer (NSCLC). They are more commonly found in adenocarcinomas, particularly in non-smokers.

- **ALK (Anaplastic Lymphoma Kinase):** This is a protein that helps control cell growth. Translation is the process of making proteins by decoding information embedded in the genetic material (messenger RNA) of any cell. Any disturbances or mutations in genes (genes are the functional units of genetic material that tell cells how to function) lead to defective protein production, which will have defective functions as well. The Anaplastic Lymphoma Kinase enzyme, which is a protein, becomes abnormal due to the ALK gene breaking off and getting attached to another gene. So, the abnormal ALK fusion protein produced starts to function abnormally and promotes cancer cell growth.

- **ROS1:** Similar to ALK, ROS1 gene fusions can drive the growth of cancer cells. These are less common but significant targets in NSCLC.

Types of Targeted Therapy

Recent breakthroughs in molecular biology have greatly improved our understanding and management of lung cancer, particularly non-small cell lung cancer (NSCLC).

As previously mentioned, EGFR mutations are among the most prevalent genetic alterations. These mutations are quite common and are present in 10-15% of lung cancer patients in Western countries and 25-30% of lung cancer patients in Asian countries. These mutations have a robust reaction to medications that target the inhibition of tyrosine kinase, which are commonly referred to as tyrosine kinase inhibitors (TKIs). EGFR TKIs have progressed through three generations, and osimertinib is now the preferred first therapy because to its better effectiveness.

ALK rearrangement and translocations are present in 2-5% of instances of non-small cell lung cancer (NSCLC). Alectinib, a second-generation TKI, is the preferable choice compared to the first-generation crizotinib. Additional ALK TKIs that have been approved include brigatinib, ceritinib, and lorlatinib.

In addition to EGFR and ALK, targeted medicines now target mutations such as ROS1 rearrangements, BRAF V600E mutations, NTRK fusions, MET exon 14 skipping, and RET rearrangements. Current research aims to broaden this list and enhance therapies for illnesses that are resistant to TKIs. These developments have greatly improved the rates of survival and the overall quality of life for individuals diagnosed with advanced non-small cell lung cancer (NSCLC).

Angiogenesis Inhibitors

Angiogenesis inhibitors target the mechanism that builds the blood supply to the tumour. By preventing the formation of new blood vessels, these drugs starve the tumour of the necessary nutrients and oxygen needed for growth. A key example is Bevacizumab (Avastin), which targets the vascular endothelial growth factor (VEGF) pathway

Monoclonal Antibodies

Monoclonal antibodies are laboratory-made molecules designed to serve as substitute antibodies that can restore, enhance, or mimic the immune system's attack on cancer cells. Cetuximab (Erbitux) is the example that targets the EGFR on cancer cells, leading to cell death.

The Effect of Targeted Therapies

Advantages

1. **Improved Survival Rates:** Targeted therapies have significantly improved survival rates, especially in patients with NSCLC who have specific genetic mutations.

2. **Minimally Adverse Effects:** These therapies target cancerous cells more precisely than normal cells, reducing side effects compared to conventional chemotherapy.

3. **Personalized Medicine:** Treatments are tailored to target individual tumour mutations, enhancing their effectiveness and providing a more personalized approach to cancer care.

Challenges

1. **Drug Resistance:** Over time, cancer cells can develop resistance to targeted therapies, necessitating the use of different drug combinations or the development of new medications.

2. **Diagnostic Requirements:** The success of targeted therapy depends on accurately identifying genetic mutations, which requires high-quality

diagnostic techniques and access to genetic testing. This can be a limitation in some settings.

Immunotherapy

Immunotherapy is a new and innovative way of treating lung cancer by enabling the patient's immune system to recognize and kill cancer cells. This approach has significantly changed the previous methods of treating the condition and provided new opportunities for patients with non-small cell lung cancer (NSCLC) and small cell lung cancer (SCLC).

The Mechanism of Immunotherapy

The core concept of immunotherapy is to stimulate the patient's own immune system against cancer cells. As a result, the patient's immune system identifies the cancer cells and eliminates them. The immune system has inherent capabilities to identify and eradicate anomalous cells, although cancer cells often acquire strategies to elude detection. Immunotherapy aims to augment the immune system's capacity to identify and eliminate cancer cells.

Types of Immunotherapies

There are several major types of immunotherapies used in lung cancer treatment:

Checkpoint Inhibitors

Checkpoint inhibitors are the drugs that target proteins on immune cells which cancer cells use to avoiding immune detection leading to rapid and uncontrollable division. By blocking these proteins, checkpoint inhibitors enable the immune system to recognize and attack cancer cells. Examples include:

- **Pembrolizumab:** Targets the PD-1 protein on immune cells.

- **Nivolumab:** Another PD-1 inhibitor.

- **Atezolizumab:** Targets the PD-L1 protein on cancer cells.

Cancer Vaccines

Cancer vaccines are designed to prompt the immune system to attack cancer cells by presenting them with specific antigens associated with these cells. Unlike traditional vaccines, which prevent disease, cancer vaccines are used to treat existing cancers by stimulating an immune response.

Adoptive Cell Therapy

Adoptive cell therapy involves taking a patient's own immune cells, modifying them in a laboratory to enhance their ability to find and kill cancer cells, and then reinfusing them into the patient. This approach has shown promise in various types of cancer, including lung cancer.

Benefits of Immunotherapy

Immunotherapy offers several benefits, particularly for lung cancer patients:

Extended Response: Immunotherapy has the potential to offer patients a more lasting response in comparison to conventional treatments. This extended response has the potential to greatly enhance patient outcomes.

Option for Patients in Advanced Stages: Immunotherapy has the potential to significantly enhance both the survival rate and overall quality of life for individuals diagnosed with advanced lung cancer. Immunotherapy has shown promise in treating patients with lung cancer metastases.

Selective Action: Immunotherapy has the remarkable ability to specifically target cancer cells, resulting in fewer side effects when compared to conventional chemotherapy and radiotherapy. Unlike these treatments, which can harm both cancerous and healthy cells, immunotherapy takes a more selective approach.

Challenges and considerations

Although immunotherapy has numerous advantages, it does have certain challenges:

Variable Response: It is challenging for doctors to determine which patients will benefit the most from immunotherapy, as not all individuals respond to this treatment. Further research and personalised treatment strategies are necessary due to the variability in response.

Side effects related to the immune system: While not as intense as the side effects of chemotherapy, certain patients may encounter immune-related side effects, where the immune system mistakenly targets healthy tissues. These symptoms may include organ inflammation, such as in the lungs, liver, or intestines.

Costs: Immunotherapy treatments can be quite costly and may be unaffordable for many individuals. The high cost may pose a barrier to accessibility and affordability for numerous patients.

The Future of Immunotherapy in Lung Cancer

The field of immunotherapy is growing rapidly, with numerous studies focusing on identifying biomarkers to help determine which patients will benefit from treatment. Research is also underway to discover new treatment targets and develop more effective therapies. This growing body of knowledge promises to make lung cancer treatment more personalized, effective, and less prone to side effects.

Ongoing Research

Researchers are continually exploring new immunotherapy approaches and combinations with other treatments to enhance efficacy and overcome resistance. With the goal of expanding the reach of immunotherapy and enhancing the well-being of patients, scientists are constantly working on the advancement of new drugs and techniques.

Personalized Medicine

Advancements in the field of personalised medicine have revolutionised healthcare. The future of immunotherapy in lung cancer lies in personalized medicine, where treatments are tailored to the specific genetic and molecular characteristics of each patient's cancer. This approach will enable more precise and effective treatments, improving survival rates and quality of life for lung cancer patients.

Chapter 10: Palliative Care in Lung Cancer

Palliative care is an essential component of lung cancer treatment, with the primary goal of enhancing the quality of life for patients. Palliative care, in contrast to curative treatments, which attempt to cure cancer, aims to ease symptoms, manage pain, and provide psychological, social, and spiritual support to the families and friends of cancer patients. The purpose of this chapter is to provide comprehensive details on palliative care in the context of lung cancer.

When it comes to individuals who have lung cancer, palliative care is really necessary, especially for those who have late stages of the disease. In palliative care, diverse patient requirements are addressed, including the management of symptoms and the maintenance of a good quality of life.

Some of the advantages of palliative care are as follows:

Symptom Relief: Symptom relief includes the management of pain, breathlessness, fatigue, and other distressing symptoms related to the disease, as well as the management of the symptoms associated with the adverse effects of medications.

- **Pain:** Often resulting from the tumour pressing on nerves or other structures. Pain management strategies include medications (analgesics, opioids), nerve blocks, and/or integrative therapies such as acupuncture and massage.

- **Breathlessness (Dyspnea):** Managed with medications (bronchodilators, steroids), oxygen therapy, and other supportive techniques.

- **Fatigue:** Addressed by improving nutrition, optimizing sleep, managing associated comorbidities, for example, anemia, and promoting physical activity within the patient's limits.

- **Cough:** Usually treated with medications such as cough suppressants and steroids.

- **Loss of Appetite and Weight Loss:** Managed through nutritional support, appetite stimulants, and dietary modifications.

Emotional and Psychological Support: Psychological care is crucial in helping patients cope with the emotional impact of lung cancer. This includes:

- **Counseling and Therapy:** Individual or group therapy sessions to address anxiety, depression, and fear.

- **Support Groups:** Connecting patients with others who are experiencing similar challenges.

- **Mind-Body Therapies:** Techniques such as meditation, mindfulness, and relaxation exercises to reduce stress and improve mental health.

Family & Social Support: Lung cancer affects not only the patient but also their family and social network.

- **Caregiver Support:** Offering guidance and assistance to family members involved in caregiving.

- **Social Services:** Assistance with practical needs such as transportation, financial issues, and accessing community resources.

- **Advance Care Planning:** Helping patients and families make informed decisions about future medical care, including advance directives and end-of-life preferences.

Spiritual Care: For many patients, spiritual well-being is an important aspect of their overall health. Its components are:

- **Spiritual Counseling:** Providing support through chaplains or spiritual advisors to address existential questions and provide comfort.

- **Cultural Sensitivity:** Respecting and incorporating the patient's cultural and religious beliefs into their care plan.

Strategies for Effective Palliative Care Implementation

Implementing efficient palliative care requires a thorough, interdisciplinary approach that emphasizes collaboration among different healthcare professionals to ensure comprehensive patient assistance. The following are the key strategies for enhancing the delivery of palliative care:

Early Integration

It is crucial to incorporate palliative care at an early stage in the treatment process in order to improve patient outcomes. Early implementation of palliative care enables proactive management of symptoms, addressing physical, emotional, and psychosocial requirements before they worsen. Early intervention not only relieves pain and discomfort, but also improves the overall quality of life, enabling patients to better manage the course of their treatment. Timely referrals to palliative care specialists guarantee that patients obtain uninterrupted, empathetic care customized to their changing requirements, leading to a substantial improvement in their overall state of health.

Utilizing a multidisciplinary team approach

An effective palliative care program relies on the cooperation of a diverse team of healthcare specialists with specialized skills and perspectives:

Physicians and nurses that specialize in areas such as palliative care, oncology, and pain management have a crucial role in developing and executing individualized care plans. Their specialized knowledge is essential in handling complicated symptoms and ensuring that the medical aspects of care are thoroughly addressed to.

Psychologists and social workers are essential in providing invaluable emotional, psychological, and social assistance. They assist patients and their families in managing the stresses and emotional difficulties that come with severe illness, promoting mental health and social welfare.

Spiritual advisors play an important part in addressing the spiritual and existential issues of patients. Spiritual counsellors provide comfort and assist individuals in discovering purpose and tranquilly amongst challenging circumstances.

Rehabilitation specialists, such as physical therapists and occupational therapists, play a crucial role in preserving and enhancing patients' functional capabilities. Their therapies facilitate patients in maintaining autonomy and enhancing their quality of life through focused physical and occupational therapy.

Effective communication and coordination

Efficient communication is the fundamental basis of well-coordinated palliative care. Consistent and open communication among the healthcare staff, patients, and their families guarantees that care plans are in sync with the patient's changing requirements and preferences. Regular meetings and updates provide prompt modifications to care strategies and guarantee full attention to all areas of the patient's condition. This collaborative approach promotes a unified care setting where all individuals are well-informed and have a shared understanding.

Education for Patients and their Families

Providing patients and their families with information and knowledge about palliative care alternatives and what to expect is essential for making well-informed decisions. By offering easily understandable written materials, informative workshops, and personalized discussions, patients and their loved ones are empowered to actively engage in the process of care planning. This educational programme aims to clarify the concept of palliative care, providing clear explanations of its advantages and procedures, thereby diminishing apprehension and promoting a feeling of autonomy and active participation in the process of care.

Surveillance and assessment

Regular and systematic monitoring and evaluation of palliative care interventions are crucial to ensure their efficacy and pinpoint areas for enhancement. Continuous evaluation using patient input, clinical outcomes, and quality of life measurements offers significant insights into the effects of healthcare. By utilizing a data-driven approach, healthcare professionals can improve and optimize care plans, guaranteeing that they remain adaptable to the patient's needs and preferences.

Chapter 11: Prehabilitation and Rehabilitation for Lung Cancer

Lung cancer is one of the most common and deadly types of cancer worldwide. Despite breakthroughs in early identification and treatment, individuals with lung cancer frequently have a poor prognosis due to the disease's aggressive nature and the major impact of treatment methods such as surgery, chemotherapy, and radiation therapy.

For the best outcomes from therapy, a comprehensive care strategy that includes both prehabilitation and rehabilitation should be adopted. This chapter explores the principles, benefits, and implementation of prehabilitation and rehabilitation in the context of lung cancer, providing a thorough understanding of how these interventions can improve patient outcomes.

Prehabilitation:

Prehabilitation is the practice of improving a patient's functional capacity prior to receiving therapy in order to enhance their physical and psychological preparedness for surgery or other therapies. Prehabilitation in lung cancer focuses on enhancing the patient's overall health condition to minimize the chances of complications during surgery, decrease the length of hospital stays, and enhance recovery after the operation.

Components of Prehabilitation

Physical Exercise

Physical activity is a fundamental component of prehabilitation for individuals with lung cancer. Customized exercise programs often consist of aerobic exercises (such as walking, cycling, or swimming), strength training (with light weights or resistance bands), and flexibility training (stretching exercises to preserve flexibility). These programs are designed to increase total physical fitness, lessen fatigue, increase muscle strength and endurance, and improve cardiovascular and pulmonary function.

Nutritional Support

Optimal nutrition is vital for patients undergoing treatment for lung cancer. Malnutrition is common in cancer patients and can adversely affect treatment outcomes. Nutritional interventions in prehabilitation include dietary assessments to identify deficiencies and create personalized nutrition plans. Protein rich diets are advised to support muscle mass and immune function in addition to supplementation with vitamins and minerals as needed.

Psychological Support

A cancer diagnosis can lead to significant psychological distress. Integrating psychological support into prehabilitation can help patients manage anxiety, depression, and stress. Interventions may include:

- Counseling or therapy sessions with a psychologist or psychiatrist.

- Mindfulness-based stress reduction techniques.

- Support groups to provide a sense of community and shared experiences.

Benefits of Prehabilitation

The benefits of prehabilitation for lung cancer patients are multifaceted. It reduces the impact of complications by improving physical fitness and nutritional status. Furthermore, it can decrease the incidence of perioperative complications such as infections and respiratory issues. Patients who are better prepared physically and mentally tend to recover more quickly after surgery or other treatments. Prehabilitation improves the overall quality of life by addressing physical, psychological, and nutritional needs before treatment.

Rehabilitation

Rehabilitation is defined by WHO as "a set of interventions designed to optimize functioning and reduce disability in individuals with health conditions in interaction with their environment". Rehabilitation involves a comprehensive approach to help patients recover and regain their functional abilities while undergoing treatment for lung cancer. It addresses the physical, psychological, and social challenges that patients may face during the recovery phase.

Components of Rehabilitation

Physical Rehabilitation

Physical rehabilitation focuses on restoring mobility, strength, and endurance. Key components include:

- **Physiotherapy:** Tailored exercises to improve respiratory function, mobility, and strength. Techniques such as deep breathing exercises and chest physiotherapy can enhance lung function.

- **Occupational Therapy:** Assistance with daily activities and strategies to improve independence and quality of life.

Nutritional Rehabilitation

Post-treatment, patients may experience side effects such as loss of appetite, taste changes, or difficulty swallowing. Nutritional rehabilitation strategies include:

- **Dietary Counseling:** Personalized plans to address specific nutritional needs and manage side effects.

- **Nutritional Supplements:** High-calorie and high-protein supplements to support recovery and prevent malnutrition.

Psychological and Emotional Support

Rehabilitation also addresses the psychological and emotional aspects of recovery. Interventions may include:

- **Counseling and Therapy:** Continued psychological support to address issues such as anxiety, depression, and post-traumatic stress.

- **Mind-Body Techniques:** Practices such as yoga, meditation, and relaxation exercises to promote mental well-being.

Benefits of Rehabilitation

Rehabilitation offers several benefits for lung cancer patients:

- **Enhanced Physical Function:** Regular exercise and physiotherapy can help restore strength, improve mobility, and reduce fatigue.

- **Improved Nutritional Status:** Addressing nutritional needs can prevent malnutrition and support overall recovery.

- **Psychological Well-being:** Ongoing psychological support can help patients cope with the emotional challenges of cancer recovery, improving overall mental health.

Implementing Prehabilitation and Rehabilitation Programs

Multidisciplinary Approach: Successful implementation of prehabilitation and rehabilitation programs requires a multidisciplinary approach involving healthcare professionals such as:

- Oncologists

- Surgeons

- Physiotherapists

- Dietitians

- Psychologists

- Occupational therapists

Personalized Care Plans

Each patient's needs are unique, necessitating personalized care plans that consider individual health status, treatment regimens, and personal preferences. A comprehensive assessment at the beginning of the prehabilitation phase can help tailor interventions to optimize outcomes. Regular monitoring and evaluation are critical to assess the effectiveness of prehabilitation and rehabilitation interventions. Adjusting care plans based on patient feedback and clinical outcomes.

In conclusion, prehabilitation and rehabilitation are essential components of comprehensive care for lung cancer patients. By addressing physical, nutritional, and psychological needs, these interventions can significantly improve treatment outcomes, enhance recovery, and improve the overall quality of life. Implementing effective prehabilitation and rehabilitation programs requires a multidisciplinary approach, personalized care plans, and continuous evaluation to ensure optimal patient care.

Chapter 12: Living with Lung Cancer

Lifestyle adjustments

Adapting to lifestyle changes is a crucial step for people with a lung cancer diagnosis to manage the condition and improve quality of life. Here, let's discuss the major lifestyle changes that can help people affected with lung cancer to improve cancer care and recovery. These include dietary changes and nutrition, physical activity, and quitting smoking.

Nutrition and Lung cancer. A healthy and balanced diet is an essential component of care and treatment for lung cancer. A balanced and healthy type of diet helps one remain strong, keep body weight at a good level, reduce the impact of any side effects relating to treatment and recover quickly.

Nutritional Needs: The metabolism of cancer and treatment can have different body demands for energy for repair and healing. Therefore, it is good for individuals to consume more proteins, vitamins, and calories and meet a dietician so that they can get a nutritional plan containing the correct type and amount of food.

Managing Side Effects: There are foods that can help reduce their common side effects like nausea, vomiting, and appetite loss. It can include consuming small, consistent foods throughout the day if you have nausea.

Supplements can be good for additional nutritional support. However, since some supplements can interfere with cancer treatment or care, it's important to contact your health professional before taking them.

Physical Activity and Lung Cancer: Regular physical activities play a crucial role in an individual's life. Walking, yoga, tai chi, can reduce fatigue, improve your mood, improve cardiovascular health, and help you perform better and adjust to healthy living better. The proper intensity and time for exercises need to be undertaken based on one's level of fitness under the guidance of a physical therapist.

Safety Considerations: It is just as important to balance physical activity with rest and avoid overexertion. Before beginning a new exercise routine, patients should consult their health care team. This is crucial if patients have bone metastasis or are vulnerable to lung infections or have cardiovascular problems.

Quitting Smoking: For people with lung cancer who smoke, this is a very important lifestyle intervention. Smoking after a lung cancer diagnosis may reduce treatment effectiveness, increase treatment side effects, and lower overall survival rates. Patients who smoke should consult with their doctor, who can guide them through smoking cessation services, counselling, or prescribing supportive drugs like nicotine replacement therapy.

Emotional and Psychological support: The diagnosis of lung cancer is associated with almost a whole gamut of emotions and psychological responses, not limited to the patient but extending to his family and loved ones. Thus, living with lung cancer is accompanied by living with emotional difficulties.

The emotional impact of lung cancer. The emotional aspect of lung cancer manifests itself by various feelings and experiences, including fear, anger, grief, and hopelessness. The image of lung cancer is strongly burdened by the patient's fear of imminent death, the choice of a treatment option, and the challenges of physical changes.

Patients can follow the following strategies to dealing with emotional issues:

- **Acknowledging and accepting**: Patients should feel that their feelings are normal during such difficult times. It is important for the patient and his family to understand that there is no one correct way to feel; individuals have a wide range of emotional responses depending on their circumstances.

- **Open conversation**: A conversation with the family, friends, or palliative care doctor about their worst fears and hopes can help in relieving themselves from stress and gain more positive attitudes. Discussing fears, treatment experiences, and how life has changed due to lung cancer helps the patient to feel supported.

- **Professional help:** Lung cancer patients may consult mental health professionals, who can provide evidence-based interventions, certain techniques, and homework assignments. Mental health professionals can help people dealing with anxiety, depression, and stress by using cognitive behavioural techniques.

- **Support Groups**: Lung cancer support groups can help patients feel less alone with their struggles. The opportunity to share experiences with others coping with a similar challenge can be both a source of relief and a valuable source of practical advice. Support groups are available in many forms, from offline meetings to online communities and social media groups.

- **Individual Counseling**: Individual counseling may be a more preferred option for a person who wants to explore their thoughts and feelings, fears, and means of dealing with them. Offering a safe space to express one's feelings, counselors can help reduce the psychological impact of living with lung cancer.

Emotional Support for Caregivers

Managing one's own emotional reactions to a lung cancer diagnosis while also meeting the physical and mental responsibilities of caregiving is a major source of emotional and psychological stress for carers. To help cope with this stress and avoid burnout, carers may benefit greatly from counselling, respite care, and support groups.

Mindfulness and Stress-Reducing Techniques

Mindfulness practices such as meditation and yoga help focus on the present moment and offer relief from feeling anxious and uncertain. These techniques can be used to cope with different lung cancer-related struggles by experiencing a state of peaceful acceptance.

Palliative Care as Part of the Emotional Support Provisions

Finally, palliative care teams fully address the physical, emotional, psychological, social, and spiritual aspects of lung cancer and they provide help to patients and as well as to their families. These professionals ensure personalized support and care at every stage of lung cancer treatment.

In conclusion, it is important to realize that every lung cancer patient also embarks on an emotional journey. By acknowledging their emotions and feelings, seeking help or joining support groups, and applying healthy coping mechanisms, patients may find ways to manage the emotional impacts of the disease.

Financial and Legal planning

A diagnosis of lung cancer can jeopardize the patient's health, social relationships, income, and the family's already shaken monthly budget. Patients and their families are ushered into the dimension of financial and legal considerations after a lung cancer diagnosis.

Understanding the financial ramifications of cancer

The cost of lung cancer is staggering; it includes surgery, chemotherapy, radiation therapy, targeted therapy, immunotherapy, hospitalization, and patient visits and readmission costs. The other costs are known as indirect costs, which involve lost income and transportation costs or remuneration for a nursing home.

Navigating insurance and medical bills Health care: Learn more about your health benefit to understand the treatments covered by your insurance premium, such as medications and care services, and learn about submitting a request and appealing if they are denied.

Cancer Support Programs: There are some medication assistance programs that can help patients pay for their medication. Some non-profit organizations can also support patients. Some doctors' offices, treatment centers, or hospitals have social workers or financial planners who can help patients identify patient assistance programs. There are several independent centers that can offer support in forms like travel support, housing support, and assistance with medical insurance. Patients can contact their healthcare team for more information on these programs.

Legal planning for the future:

An advance directive is a legal document that may include a living will and medical power of attorney. A living will spell out particular types of medical care and life-extending interventions that you wish or do not wish in case you become severely or terminally sick and are unable to communicate your desires. The healthcare power of the attorney names a trusted person to make healthcare decisions on your behalf if you become incapacitated.

Chapter 13: Prevention of Lung Cancer

Cancers that can be prevented to a large extent include lung cancer. Although it is not possible to completely eliminate the risk of developing lung cancer, following a healthy lifestyle can considerably lessen the likelihood of having the condition. Reducing exposure to carcinogens, quitting smoking, and keeping a healthy lifestyle are the primary focuses of prevention methods. All three of these key preventative measures will be discussed in depth in this chapter.

Quitting Smoking:

The Impact of Cigarette Smoking: Approximately 85% of lung cancer cases can be attributed to cigarette smoking. The incidence of lung cancer is directly proportional to both the quantity of cigarettes consumed and the total duration of smoking. Individuals who engage in smoking are subject to a notably elevated level of risk in comparison to those who do not smoke. However, it is encouraging to note that quitting smoking can substantially diminish this risk over a period of time.

Advantages of Smoking Cessation: Quitting smoking leads to a substantial reduction in the likelihood of acquiring lung cancer. Research has demonstrated that the likelihood of developing lung cancer reduces by around 50% after a decade of cessation in comparison to individuals who continue smoking.

Methods for Cessation of Smoking: Successfully quitting smoking often necessitates a comprehensive approach that encompasses:

- Counseling that includes behavioural treatment. It can assist people in comprehending their smoking triggers and adopting techniques to control their cravings for cigarettes.

- Drugs, such as varenicline and bupropion can also advised by health professionals when needed to effectively alleviate cravings and withdrawal symptoms associated with quitting smoking.

- Nicotine Replacement Therapy (NRT): Nicotine patches, gums, lozenges, and inhalers are the different types of NRTs. They can be consumed at regulated amount to decrease the dependency on cigarettes and alleviate withdrawal symptoms.

- Support Groups: Support groups offer emotional support and encouragement from individuals who are also striving to quit.

Healthcare professionals can provide tailored approaches and tools to assist clients in quitting smoking, greatly enhancing their likelihood of achieving success.

Lowering Radon Risk

As was discussed in earlier chapters, Radon is a radioactive gas produced by the natural decay of uranium in rocks and soils and is the second most common cause of lung cancer development after smoking. It is not possible to sense the presence of this gas in our surroundings with our natural senses since it is an odourless, colourless, and tasteless gas.

To lower the risk of exposure, anyone can seek assistance from radon testing services. Besides, there are radon test kits available that can be used to assess the levels. If high levels of radon are detected, radon mitigation systems can be installed to reduce radon concentrations. These systems typically involve venting radon gas from beneath the building to the outside, preventing it from accumulating indoors.

Reducing Contact with Carcinogens

Occupational and Environmental Carcinogens: Workplace exposure to known carcinogens such as asbestos, arsenic, chromium, and nickel is one of the most important risk factors for developing lung cancer as well as other types of cancer. If proper precautions are not taken at workplaces, the minimal everyday exposures can significantly increase the risk of developing lung cancer. Therefore, people who may get exposed to any carcinogens at their workplaces must follow occupational safety and health regulations to minimize such hazardous exposures. Both employers and employees must adhere to safety norms and standards to minimize the risk.

Key strategies can include:

- **Personal Protective Equipment (PPE):** Using masks, gloves, and protective clothing can reduce direct contact with carcinogens.

- **Ventilation:** Ensuring adequate ventilation in workspaces can help disperse harmful substances.

- **Monitoring:** Regular monitoring of air quality and contaminant levels can help detect and mitigate risks promptly.

Maintaining a Healthy Routine

Nutrition: Diet has a very significant role in keeping anyone healthy and devoid of diseases. The correlation of cancer development with unhealthy food items has clearly been established in research. Following are some unhealthy items that should be avoided as much as possible to keep ourselves away from cancer.

- **Reducing Processed and Red Meat:** High consumption of processed meats (e.g., bacon, sausages) and red meats has been linked to an increased risk of several cancers, including lung cancer.

- **Limiting Alcohol Consumption:** Alcohol is a known carcinogen, and its consumption should be moderated or avoided to reduce cancer risk.

- **Avoiding High-Fat and High-Sugar Foods:** These foods contribute to obesity, which is a risk factor for many cancers.

- **Eating a Plant-Based Diet:** A diet rich in fruits, vegetables, whole grains, and legumes provides fiber, vitamins, and antioxidants that can help protect against cancer.

Exercise: Regular exercise provides several benefits, including its impact on lowering the risk of developing cancer. Physical activity not only helps maintain an ideal weight and body mass index but also improves immune function and reduces inflammation. 30 minutes of physical activity (walking, cycling, swimming, or even gardening) can be very beneficial to keeping anyone physically and mentally healthy.

Addressing Air Pollution: With increasing industrialization and the number of vehicles on the roads, air pollution is increasing rapidly. Research has found several hazardous elements in polluted air that can cause lung cancer in people who are significantly exposed to them. The very small, invisible, and hazardous suspended particles in the air, also known as particulate matter, can reach directly to our alveoli and get deposited into them, eventually leading to DNA damage and malignancy. All possible efforts must be made to reduce air pollution and its exposure to us. Following is some of the strategies that can be followed in order to reduce exposure and the risk of lung cancer:

- **Monitor Air Quality:** Keep track of air quality indices and avoid outdoor activities during high pollution days.

- **Stay Indoors:** During peak pollution times, stay indoors and use air purifiers to improve indoor air quality.

- **Wear Masks:** When outdoor activities are unavoidable, wearing masks can help filter out harmful particles.

Wellness Preventive Services

Regular Checkups

It is a good practice to go for regular health checkups, especially for those who are smokers or exposed to carcinogens in any form. Regular checkups give an opportunity to catch any developing diseases early, which may be prevented from progressing further by early and effective interventions. These checkups can also identify any potential risk factors in our bodies that might increase the risk of lung cancer development. You can always book an appointment and discuss with your healthcare providers any issues that you think may be a risk factor for any serious disease in the future. Remember, prevention, early detection, and timely intervention are the keys to stopping any disease from developing or worsening.

Screening Programs

Screening programmes for high-risk individuals, such as chronic and heavy smokers, can be lifesaving. As we have already discussed in previous chapters, low dose computed tomography (LDCT) scans are very effective in detecting lung cancer at an early stage without causing any significant radiation exposure during the screening process. You can consult your healthcare professionals, who can help determine your eligibility for lung cancer screening.

In summary, preventing lung cancer involves a multifaceted approach that includes quitting smoking, reducing exposure to carcinogens, maintaining a healthy lifestyle, and utilizing preventive health services. While it is not always possible to eliminate the risk entirely, these strategies can significantly lower the chances of developing lung cancer. By understanding and implementing these preventive measures, individuals can take proactive steps to protect their health and reduce the burden of lung cancer. Living with lung cancer requires ongoing management and support, but taking preventive measures can make a substantial difference in outcomes. Educating the public about these strategies and promoting healthy behaviors are crucial steps in the fight against lung cancer.

Chapter 14: The Future of Lung Cancer Research and Treatment

Lung cancer continues to be the leading cause of death from cancer on a global scale, presenting significant challenges to healthcare systems worldwide. Nevertheless, progress in scientific investigation and medical care during the last decade has resulted in enhanced results and new hope for patients. This chapter explores the future of lung cancer research and treatment, focusing on developing technology, novel medicines, and the possible influence of personalised medicine.

Advances in Early Detection and Screening

Liquid Biopsies

Liquid biopsies, unlike traditional biopsies that require tissue samples, analyze circulating tumour DNA (ctDNA) in the blood. This novel method represents a promising advancement in the early detection of lung cancer. This non-invasive method allows for early detection by identifying genetic mutations and biomarkers associated with lung cancer at an early stage. It allows monitoring of disease progression and response to ongoing treatment by regularly analyzing blood samples. Research into liquid biopsies is rapidly evolving, with ongoing studies aiming to improve their sensitivity and accuracy.

Improved Imaging Techniques

Advanced technologies are improving imaging techniques and their quality, which benefit us by enhancing the accuracy of the detection of lung cancer and its staging. For instance, molecular imaging techniques such as positron emission tomography (PET) scans combined with CT or MRI can provide detailed images of cancerous tissues and assess metabolic activity. These advancements are expected to lead to earlier diagnosis and improved survival rates.

Personalized Medicine and Targeted Therapies

With advancements in genomic profiling, the management of lung cancer has been completely transformed. Genomic profiling provides comprehensive and precise data, which allows for a more individualised approach in the management of lung cancer. With the power of Next-Generation Sequencing (NGS), we can now analyse multiple genes at once to uncover mutations that can be effectively targeted with medicines (targeted therapies). Many drugs have already been developed to target specific genetic mutations in lung cancer. Some examples are EGFR inhibitors, ALK inhibitors, etc.

Similarly, immunotherapy is also a fascinating new field that holds great promise in the treatment of various diseases, including lung cancer. Immunotherapy has emerged as a groundbreaking treatment for lung cancer, harnessing the body's immune system to fight cancer cells. Checkpoint Inhibitors, such as pembrolizumab and nivolumab, inhibit the functions of proteins that inhibit the immune cells' ability to attack cancer cells.

Advances in Radiotherapy

Stereotactic Body Radiotherapy (SBRT), that delivers high doses of radiation with pinpoint accuracy to small, well-defined tumours have several benefits, for example minimizing damage to surrounding healthy tissues, requiring fewer treatment sessions compared to conventional radiotherapy.

Proton Therapy

The proton beam therapy, often known as PBT, is a form of radiation therapy that uses proton particles rather than x-rays to administer radiation. Due to the fact that protons possess certain physical properties, the amount of radiation that is deposited in the normal tissue that is located beyond the tumour is substantially lower. Due to these properties PBT delivers maximum radiation dose directly to the tumour while sparing nearby healthy tissues and lowers the risk of radiation-induced damage to surrounding organs and tissues. Research into optimizing proton therapy protocols is ongoing, with the goal of expanding its accessibility and effectiveness.

Precision Surgery

Robotic-assisted surgeries for the management of lung cancer significantly enhance the precision of surgeries. These surgeries are minimally invasive, characterized by smaller incisions, reduced pain, and faster recovery times, and they have greater precision in tumour removal.

Emerging Therapies

Epigenetic Therapies and Nanotechnology

Epigenetic therapies specifically focus on the chemical alterations that control gene expression, while leaving the DNA sequence unchanged. These medicines seek to reprogram cancer cells by restoring their normal function through undoing abnormal epigenetic alterations. In addition, epigenetic medicines have the potential to improve the effectiveness of current treatments, such as chemotherapy and immunotherapy. Although research into epigenetic drugs is still in its early stages, preliminary results are promising.

Nanotechnology provides novel methods for the treatment of lung cancer. Targeted drug delivery is a strategy that involves using nanoparticles to directly deliver medications to cancer cells, resulting in improved effectiveness and decreased adverse effects. Another potential use is early diagnosis, where nanosensors have the ability to identify cancer biomarkers at extremely low levels. In addition, theranostics, a method that integrates therapy and diagnostics into a single platform, enables the continuous monitoring of treatment response in real-time.

Tumour Microenvironment Modulation

The tumour microenvironment plays a crucial role in cancer progression and response to treatment. Future therapies aim to disrupt tumour support systems by targeting the blood vessels, immune cells, and other components that support tumour growth. Additionally, modifying the tumour microenvironment to make it more susceptible to immune attack can enhance the immune response, providing a more effective strategy for combating lung cancer.

Conclusion

The future of lung cancer research and treatment is filled with promise and potential. Advances in early detection, personalized medicine, immunotherapy, radiotherapy, and emerging technologies such as nanotechnology are paving the way for more effective and less invasive treatments. As research continues to evolve, a more comprehensive, patient-centered approach to lung cancer care is becoming possible and is offering hope and improved outcomes for patients worldwide.